MAGNETIC Therapy

healing in your hands

ABBOT GEORGE BURKE

DeVorss & Company
P.O. BOX 550, Marina del Rey, CA 90294-0550

First DeVorss & Co. Edition, 1987

Second Printing, 1988

0-87516-588-5

Illustrations by Bro. Simeon Davis

Library of Congress Cataloging in Publication Data
Burke, George, 1940-
    Magnetic therapy.

    Bibliography: p.
    1. Magnetic healing.   2. Animal magnetism.
I. Title.
RZ422.B87   615.8'45   80-22941

Printed in the United States of America

TABLE OF CONTENTS

MAGNETIC THERAPY

1

WHAT IS MAGNETISM AND MAGNETIC THERAPY?

Two hundred years ago the great healer, Dr. Franz Anton Mesmer, wrote: "All doubts have been removed from my mind that there exists in Nature a universally acting principle which, independently of ourselves, operates—and which we vaguely attribute to Art *and* Nature."

If I gave you a neatly packaged definition of Magnetism I would simply be putting you on. Such a thing cannot be produced for two reasons: (1) limitation of study of the question, and (2) limitation of our knowledge of the forces circulating around us in the universe. This much I can tell you: it is a force, a power. And this force/power behaves like electricity (whatever *that* really is) and magnetism (ditto). Many people have thought it is much more, some attributing even Divinity to it, and others have considered it to be much less. Some think it does not exist at all except in the power of suggestion (whatever that is, as well). But most people just don't have any idea about it at all because they have never heard or thought of it.

Historical Views On Magnetism

The great German poet-philosopher, Goethe, said: "Magnetism is a universal active power, which everyone possesses, differing only according to his individuality. Its effects extend to everything and in all cases. The Magnetic power of man reaches out to all mankind, to animals and to plants."

The philosopher Schopenhauer was even more firm: "Whoever doubts the fact of healing Magnetism is not only unbelieving but ignorant."

Many inscriptions and figures on ancient Egyptian tablets show definitely that the Egyptians were accustomed to using Magnetism for healing the sick.

Among the ancients, Aesculapius was considered the founder of the healing art. And his name is sworn by in the Hippocratic Oath taken by all modern American physicians. Yet we are told by the ancient writings that Aesculapius healed mostly through the application of Magnetism to

1

the suffering.

Therefore the Flemish philosopher, Von Helmont, wrote: "Magnetism is active everywhere, and has nothing new but the name: it is a paradox only to those who ridicule whatever they themselves are unable to explain."

Celsus, nearly two thousand years ago, was a vigorous advocate of this form of Magnetic treatment, and incidentally proves that it was known and practiced long before his time.

Magnetism was daily practiced in the temples of Isis, Osiris, and Serapis. In these temples the priests treated the sick and cured them, mostly with Magnetism, imparted in various ways. Mummy cases and talismans, as well as wall paintings, show priests and priestesses treating the sick with varying positions of the hands. All such representations were a "mystery" only to those unacquainted with Magnetism and its techniques of application.

In February of 1826, a commission was appointed by the French Government to study the "case" of Magnetic Therapy. For five years the members studied the application and effects of Magnetism and finally drew up their report in 1831. At the end of the document thirty "conclusions" were enumerated, the twenty-ninth being: "Considered as a cause of certain psychological phenomena, or as a therapeutic remedy, Magnetism ought to be allowed a place within the circle of medical sciences."

A Personal View

My opinion is that what I am calling Magnetism in this book is electricity, magnetism, and quite a lot more. Mesmer called it "Animal Magnetism." By "animal" he meant soul (in Latin: *anima*) power, that fundamental life-force which animates all living bodies. Others called it "Vital Magnetism," but really meant the same things, because "vital" comes from the Latin word *vita*—life.

"And God . . . breathed upon his face the breath of life, and the man became a living soul" (Genesis 2:7). The word translated "soul" here is *psychin* (psyche), which means much more than spirit—it means the whole living complex of a human being, especially his mind. And since the ruling power of the mind over our bodies has been more than adequately demonstrated by modern psychology in its studies of psychosomatic disease, we can see that this particular term is perfect in expressing the origin of life in man. Modern physics has definitely established that the life which is in man is also in the entire universe. Here, too, the Genesis account has something to say: "And God said, Let there be light, and there was" (Genesis 1:3), long before the suns lit up the universe. When

2

Paramhansa Yogananda—known to millions through his *Autobiography of a Yogi*—visited the Bavarian stigmatist and miracle-worker, Theresa Neumann, in 1935, he asked her how it was possible for her to have lived for years (when she passed away in 1962, it was nearly *forty* years!) without food or drink of any kind whatsoever. The following is his account:

"'Den't you eat anything?' I wanted to hear the answer from her own lips.

"'No, except a Host [Communion wafer] at six o'clock each morning.'

"'How large is the Host?'

"'It is paper-thin, the size of a small coin.' She added, 'I take it for sacramental reasons; if it is unconsecrated, I am unable to swallow it.'

"'Certainly you could not have lived on that, for twelve whole years?'

"'I live by God's light.'

"How simple her reply, how Einsteinian!

"'I see you realize that energy flows to your body from the ether, sun, and air.'

"A swift smile broke over her face. 'I am so happy to know you understand how I live.'"

In other words, putting the biblical account and this modern narrative together, we can see that "light" signifies the fundamental life-force in all things, *and its various modifications* in the varying forms of existence.

"An illuminating experiment was made by Lafontaine with a number of lizards. They were deprived of all food. Two of the lizards were treated by magnetic strokings, the fingers being held just above the skin as they travelled down the body. Those lizards that were not so treated died for want of nourishment, while those two which received the strokings along their bodies outlived the others, one by forty-two days and the other by seventy-five days, still without food." (Leslie O. Korth, *Healing Magnetism*, p. 19)

From my observation it seems evident that what I am calling Magnetism is a single entity, but it has many aspects and manifestations. It is indeed electrical and magnetic; but it is much more.

In the Sankhya system of ancient East Indian physics, this fundamental life-force was called *prana*, which literally means just that—"life-force." However, the Sankhya system postulates that there are five major types or modifications of *prana*: these in turn are subdivided into subtler modifications according to required functions in universal life, and these again can be multiplied by two, since there are positive and negative aspects of all energies. And each of these has a name. Let's just use one!

3

When a car passes us on the street we don't say: "There goes a chassis, engine, battery, gas tank, drive shaft, transmission, etc., etc., down the street." We just use a name for the whole complex thing and say it is an automobile; a car. Which is reasonable, since it functions as a unit to accomplish its function of getting us someplace. And similarly the life-force functions harmoniously in its various aspects to get us through our cycle of life. I personally like the term Magnetism, inadequate as it may be technically. But it is not inaccurate. You can put any name to it you like in your working with it—but do put it to work! Magnetism by any other name is just as powerful and beneficial. And just as necessary to learn about and use.

"Vital Force is that which underlies all physical action of the body. It is that which causes the circulation of the blood—the movements of the cells—in fact all the motions upon which depend the life of the physical body. Without this Vital Force, there could be no life—no motion—no action. Some call it 'nervous force,' but it is the one thing, no matter by what name it may be called. It is this force· that is sent forth from the nervous system by an effort of the will, when we wish a muscle to move. . . .

"Man absorbs his supply of Vital Force from the food he eats; the water he drinks; and largely from the air he breathes. . . . This Vital Energy is stored up in the Brain, and great nerve centres of the body, from which it is drawn to supply the constantly arising wants of the system. It is distributed over the wires of the nervous system, to all parts of the body. In fact, every nerve is constantly charged with Vital Force, which is replenished when exhausted. Every nerve is a 'live wire,' through which the flow of Vital Force proceeds. And, more than this, every cell in the body, no matter where it is located, or what work it is doing, contains more or less Vital Energy, at all times.

"A strong, healthy person is one who is charged with a goodly supply of Vital Force, which travels to all parts of the body, refreshing, stimulating, and producing activity and energy. Not only does it do this, but it surrounds his body like an aura, and may be felt by those coming in contact. A person depleted of Vital Force will manifest ill-health, lack of vitality, etc., and will only regain his normal condition when he replenishes his store of Vitality." So says William Walker Atkinson.

Without planning to, I have already told you what it does (so much for my carefully thought-out outline for this book!): it flows throughout the universe, enlivening all things. This is why Mesmer also called it "vital fluid." Don't confuse fluid with liquid, like the old Greek philosopher,

4

Thales, who claimed that all things were made of water. Water it is not, but fluid it is. In fact, the substance of the whole universe is the same, whether it manifests as solid, liquid, gas, or what-have-you. But one fundamental aspect or form of that substance is the "mechanic" of creation as well as its "fuel." And *that* we are calling "Magnetism." This force moves invisibly through all existing things, maintaining that process which we call "life," no matter how vague our ideas or definitions of that may be. And that force can flow in basically two ways: harmoniously or inharmoniously; rhythmically or sporadically; freely or obstructed to some degree. When it becomes totally blocked or reduced to below a critical degree the result is death.

So we can say that harmonious, unobstructed flow of this Magnetism is health. Inharmonious or obstructed flow of Magnetism is disease. And the cessation of Magnetic flow or its critical reduction results in death. (Though nothing ever really dies—it only changes. Both Spirit and Matter are alive; but Spirit does not change, and Matter does.) Mesmer put it this way: "Man is in a condition of health when all parts of which he is composed are able to exercise the functions for which they were destined. If perfect order rules all of his functions, one calls this state the state of harmony. Sickness is the opposite state—that is, one wherein harmony is disturbed. . . . The remedy is that which reestablishes the order or harmony which has been disturbed." And again: "Life in all creatures in the universe is one and the same: it consists of the movement of the most subtle substance. Death is repose, or the cessation of motion. The natural and inevitable course of life consists in passing through the state of fluidity to that of solidity. . . . Illness is therefore nothing more than a disturbance of the progression of the movement of life."

More modern research has also come to the same conclusions. Sister Justa Smith, enzymologist and chairman of the chemistry department at Rosary Hill College in Buffalo, New York, has been deeply studying the effect of the healing forces—emanating from the hands—on enzymes. She has established that magnetic fields increase enzyme activity, while ultraviolet light damages it. Not only did Sister Justa find that the enzymes were greatly increased in activity when held in the hands of a magnetically strong person, she also discovered that if she damaged enzymes with ultraviolet light and then had that vial held in the same person's hands for some time, the enzymes would be "healed"—restored to their normal activity. Further, she also experimented with exposing enzymes to high magnetic fields using regular magnets. She found that the activity of the enzymes in the vial treated by the healer was the same as the vials subjected to a magnetic field of thirteen thousand gauss!

You Are A Magnet

Man himself is a magnet. From the moment of his conception this universal Magnetism begins to flow through his physical entity until its cessation at his death. This reveals another principle: by its presence the *spirit* stimulates this flow we call life, and by its departure that flow ceases. In other words, the spirit causes this flow which in turn causes the life of the body. As God the Universal Spirit causes life in all matter, so the individual spirit causes the microcosm of the body to live and function in the greater universe.

Proof that everything is alive is that everything is *magnetic*. There is nothing in existence that does not have two poles—positive and negative. In testing a piece of string, even, one end will be found positive and the other negative. Cut it, and each piece will be found to have the two poles. Chop the string into dozens of pieces—each fragment will test out as having two poles. Break a twig from a tree, and you will find the same thing. This page you are reading is the same, also.

Animals have even more magnetism. Some time ago in Lima, Peru, there was a colony of termites which discharged electric currents of such intensity that the short-wave reception in their vicinity was disturbed. The Lima fire brigade had to be called out to destroy the termites.

But your body is a much more powerful magnet, your two hands being its major poles. Subtle Magnetism is flowing within them constantly. Your touching of this page is charging it with that Magnetism. Anything you touch becomes to some degree magnetized. A very sensitive person can detect this Magnetism, and that we call psychometry—nothing mysterious or supernatural about it at all. If you can project a very intense and grosser type of this Magnetism from your hands or head (through the eyes) it is psychokinetic force. This is how "psychics" bend spoons, stop watches, etc.; and how Nelya Mikhailova, the Soviet psychokineticist made known through *Psychic Discoveries Behind the Iron Curtain*, can move objects—especially metal ones, which are the most sensitive to Magnetism—by moving her hands over them.

Your body is a magnet, as I have said, but that is oversimplifying things. It is really several magnets hooked together to act as one. The human body can be pictured as four magnets: three horseshoe magnets and one bar magnet. Your two feet are the poles of one horseshoe, your hands are the poles of another, and the right and left sides of your head are the third (the eyes being the projectors of that Magnetic force). The

6

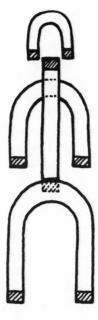

Fig. 1

spine is connecting these three, running through the middle of the body as a bar magnet—its two ends being the two poles (see Fig. 1).

In this century we have "gadget craze," and a multitude of healing machines of all types, some accepted by the medical profession and some not, have been invented and patented. But the perfect therapeutic apparatus, the true "healing machine," is your own body. "Therefore, of all the bodies, the one which can act most effectively upon man is his fellow-man," concluded Mesmer. Through your two hands that machine can be operated to restore health to yourself and others. Why? Because health is a harmonious, unobstructed flow of the life-force, and your hands can stimulate that life-force to flow through the body in a free and balanced way so the body can heal itself. Each person's body is the healer. You will never heal. Rather, the natural life-force whose flow you will increase or balance will do the healing. There is no other healer in the natural order of things. Even Divine, supernatural healing is a restoration and regularization of that force. The same is true of medicine. Medicine only facilitates the body's self-repairing capacity. No matter what a medical doctor, osteopath, chiropractor, naturopath, or herbalist prescribes, they are all one in the final analysis: life-force regulators.

Dr. A.S. Raleigh's analysis is thus: "We speak of heart disease, for instance, but as a matter of fact, we do not mean that the heart is diseased. Were anything to get wrong with the heart organically, the patient would not last very long. What we mean by heart disease is a weakened or disturbed condition of the cardiac nerve center, which causes the heart to get out of gear in the sense that the proper quantity of nervous stimuli is not communicated to the heart. The result is, the heart is not able to perform its functions; thus we say it is diseased; that is, it is out of harmony, so with all the other diseases that are to be included under the functional head.

"We should conceive of an organ or muscle as being a machine, a motor,

7

in fact, or rather, a machine run by a motor. The nerve center controlling this organ or muscle is the motor that runs the machine. Now, the analogy is perfect between the nerve center and the motor in ordinary machines; if the motor receives a proper quantity of electricity it will run the machine in the proper manner. . . . If the current of nervous stimuli flowing over the sympathetic nervous system and reaching the nerve center governing those organs, be normal, if the equilibrium be maintained, perfect health in those functions will be the result; each nerve center will receive a sufficient quantity of Prana to enable it to compel the organ to perform its proper functions. But if the current be weak or too strong or spasmodic, a corresponding result will take place. . . .

"Any method which will restore the equilibrium in the circulation of the nerve force will cure any functional disease in the world. You may benefit the condition by applying nervous stimuli direct to the nerve center controlling the organ. Magnetic Healing has, therefore, been found of very much value in the treatment of functional diseases, because they give the nerve force for which that nerve center is starving. Giving this nerve force, they establish the equilibrium, they strengthen the organ or rather the nerve center, so that it makes the organ perform its proper functions. . . .

"There is no disease of a functional character to which flesh is heir, that cannot be cured by this method and cured with comparative ease. There is no functional disease that can be cured permanently in any other way. Even those medicines such as arsenic and actina that are given by physicians, are really given for the purpose of accomplishing this result, by causing a certain stimulus to be imparted to the nerve centers in an artificial manner which will thus draw to them the nervous force.

"Remember, therefore, that in our method of healing we are employing the same fundamental principle that all intelligent physicians employ. Our methods are, of course, a little more scientific, they are more fundamental than theirs, but it is not a new departure, it is not a new fad, it is simply the application of the old physiological method of removing the cause and allowing Nature to take care of itself."

Once an osteopath was asked, while giving a treatment, what he was trying to accomplish, to which he replied, "I am releasing the life forces."

Magnetic Therapy is the most basic and direct way of effecting that life-force, which we call Magnetism. And it has great advantages:

(1) It can increase the flow of life-force into the body for general good health. Sickness need not be the motivation for Magnetic treatment.

To live, the body must not only have a free circulation of life-force, it

8

must have an *inflowing* of it from the world around it. Normally, this life-power enters the body through the feet, hands, and head. But if the body weakens in its magnetism—just as a magnet can become weakened—the supply of life-force is cut down to a level below that "voltage" needed for correct operation, and the magnetically starved (or "suffocating") body becomes ill. Magnetic Therapy immediately increases the influx of vital power in the body and remagnetizes it, thus revitalizing its natural magnetic power of drawing life-force into itself. This is why Mesmer could state with such confidence: "It will be established from the facts, according to the rules which I will set forth, that Animal Magnetism will cure, immediately, all diseases of the nerves, and, mediately, all other diseases."

(2) Magnetic Therapy can right away stimulate the supply and flow of life-force to a troubled area that has become vitality-starved through some obstruction. And in the increase of flow the obstruction is ultimately removed, just as a clogged water pipe can be cleared by flushing it out with an increased flow of water.

(3) Some diseases are a result of a leaking out of the vital force from the body, just as holes in a gas tank will cause a lack of fuel. Magnetic Therapy restores the normal channels of flow in the life-force and, in effect, "seals" the leaks.

(4) Everything is divided into positive and negative, and the life-force is no exception. It, too, can become negative, disturbed, inert—even, we might say, diseased. Negative life-force accumulating in the body, especially through a blockage of this life-force's flow, can cause ill-health in the same way continual breathing of stale or foul air can cause devitalization and even illness. If it becomes localized, an organ becomes impaired in in its operation or even damaged. What is poison? It is any substance which imparts an energy or operation to the body that destroys its natural harmony and is antithetical to its normal functioning. So also, subtle life-force can be poison to the body and its organs. Magnetic Therapy can remove this toxic magnetism in a very direct way.

(5) Even if the flow of life-force is unobstructed, there will be problems if it is not flowing in the right channels—that is, if the polarity is confused, and the Magnetism is not flowing from the negative to the positive poles of the body as it should. Conflict in the Magnetic flow develops blockages, leaks, and deficiencies—in other words: *disease*. Magnetic Therapy corrects polarity as the first step in its application, whereas this vital aspect of of health is ignored in nearly all other systems of medicine and therapy.

Does this mean that Magnetic Therapy is a cure-all? *Not at all!* Magnetic Therapy does not cure; it simply aids the body to cure itself by

9

supplying it with curative force. Nor should other modes of treatment be abandoned. Your body needs all the help it can get in this radioactive, polluted world of ours. But I do believe that Magnetic Therapy is an invaluable aid to health. Why?

First, it operates right at the heart of the disease—the life-force.

Second, it requires no diagnosis or prescribing of medicine or physical therapy.

Third, the only knowledge you need is that found in the practical principles of application which are given in this book. And they are so simple that once you learn them well you can forget this book forever. Remember: this system is *therapy*, not *medicine*. Knowledge of disease and its medicinal treatment is irrelevant to the application of Magnetic Therapy. Medicinal treatment of disease is the domain of trained doctors (of whatever school of medicine), and should not be trespassed upon.

Fourth, no tools are needed. Just your hands.

Fifth, everybody can do it.

Can you get more fundamental and universal than that? Magnetic Therapy stands on the broadest base of all: *Life*.

"Experience alone will scatter the clouds and shed light on this important truth: that NATURE AFFORDS A UNIVERSAL MEANS OF HEALING AND PRESERVING MEN"—Dr. Franz Anton Mesmer.

How is Magnetic Therapy applied? In the simplest way possible: by the application of the hands as poles of a magnet in order to increase and normalize the flow of life-force in your body and those of others.

Enough words! Let's get down to the "how-to" of it.

2

hOW TO dO IT

First, get acquainted with yourself as a magnet. As I said before, your body is a great magnet composed of several magnets. But it is simple to formulate:

If You Are Right-Handed

(1) Your right hand, your right foot, the right side of your head, and the entire right side of your body are *positive*.

(2) Your left hand, your left foot, the left side of your head, and the entire left side of your body are *negative*.

If You Are Left-Handed

(1) Your left hand, your left foot, the left side of your head, and the entire left side of your body are *positive*.

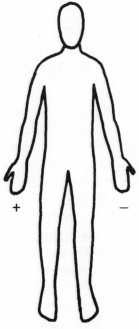

Fig. 2 - Right-Handed

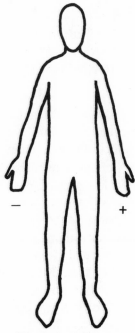

Fig. 3 - Left-Handed

(2) Your right hand, your right foot, the right side of your head, and the entire right side of your body are *negative*.

For Both Types of Handedness

In *both* right-handed and left-handed people, the spine is positive at the top and negative at the bottom (see Fig. 4).

Principles in Brief

Anyhow, you will be working with your hands only, so all you really need to remember is:

(1) If you are right-handed, your *right* hand is *positive* and your *left* hand is *negative* (see Fig. 2).

(2) If you are left-handed, your *left* hand is *positive* and your *right* hand is *negative* (see Fig. 3).

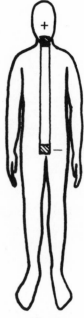

Fig. 4

To Simplify

To avoid confusion and multiplication of words, I will only be using the terms "negative hand" and "positive hand" in the instructions. So it is important to memorize the above according to your handedness.

Getting Ready

As you know, most magnets are metal, since that substance is the most easily magnetized. And we have all heard (or seen) that a steel needle when rubbed by a magnet becomes a magnet itself temporarily. The principle: *metal attracts and absorbs Magnetism.* Therefore metal can hinder the Magnetic flow where it contacts the body, either making it accumulate in just one spot rather than flow evenly, or it can draw it off from the body, causing a "leak." So the first step in applying Magnetism to yourself or others is to see that neither you nor the recipient are wearing any metal (jewelry, wristwatches, etc.), as this can interfere with the Magnetic flow. Rings apparently do not effect Magnetism, however, and need not be removed. I myself always wear a light metal chain with a small metal crucifix and a St. Benedict medal attached to it, and it has not interfered with my Magnetic work. But ordinary chains, necklaces, bracelets, etc., should be removed before attempting Magnetic Therapy. Later on, when you are able to sense for yourself the Magnetic flow, you can experiment to see whether some of your jewelry can be worn without cutting down the Magnetic flow. But for now, be safe and remove it all.

During Magnetic Therapy, neither you nor the recipient should be touching metal. If the recipient will be sitting, be sure that the chair is not metal, or that the recipient is not touching any metal ornamentation on a non-metal chair. If the recipient is lying on a bed with a metal frame, be sure he is not touching it in any way or that you are not accidentally touching your leg against it while bending over him. A layer of cloth (except for wool or silk) between will not insulate you or the recipient enough.

Also, neither you nor the recipient should be wearing wool or silk, as that insulates against Magnetism. Later, when you are proficient in detecting the subtleties of the Magnetic flow you may want to test whether certain man-made, synthetic fibers might not also hinder the Magnetic effect. Moreover, neither of you should be wearing leather belts or shoes, as this really blocks the Magnetic flow. I will talk more about this later. Leather "clothes" are a hindrance also, and should be removed for Magnetic Therapy.

During the therapy the recipient should not have legs or arms crossed, his hands or feet touching one another, one of his hands touching the opposite arm or leg, or one of his feet touching the opposite leg.

If sitting for the therapy, the recipient should sit with feet flat on the floor, and his hands resting on his thighs (unless that interferes with you reaching a spot that needs treatment).

If lying down for the therapy, the recipient should lie flat on his back, or on his stomach, with his arms relaxed at his side—but his hands not touching his body—and his legs straight out and slightly separated so his feet do not touch each other.

Never should the recipient touch the operator or vice versa. Be sure that if you have to lean over the recipient you are not touching his body in any way. Otherwise a circuit will be formed that will interfere with the Magnetic flow.

How Magnetic Are You?

Now let's find out how magnetic you are. Although I believe that there is no normal, healthy person who cannot successfully apply Magnetism, there is no doubt that there are varying degrees of magnetic intensity in people—that is, in some people the Magnetism is flowing much stronger than in others, and therefore their treatment will be more effective and rapid in its results.

How To Find Out

Here is the method to check your own magnetic strength.

Correct your polarity first (see page 16). Then hold your two hands with the palms facing each other about eight inches apart (see Fig. 5). Just relax and concentrate on how your palms *feel*. You may need to wait for a while (even a few minutes) before you do feel anything, but that is all right. If you are magnetic enough to begin practicing this therapy, you should after a while feel a

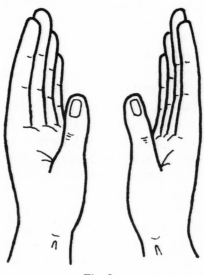

Fig. 5

tingling, "electric" sensation in your palms, or a sensation that they are being drawn together or repelled from one another like magnets, or a feeling of heat or cold, or even the sensation of having a ball or balloon pressing your palms slightly between the hands.

If this method does not "work" for you—does not indicate that you are highly magnetic—do not be discouraged. Instead, read the chapter on Increasing Your Magnetism, and apply what is found there as far as is practical for you. Especially try to get some copper rings as described there. They usually increase anyone's Magnetism sufficiently for this practice.

The Five Methods

Basically there are only five things to learn:
(1) Polarity Correction
(2) Body Sweep
(3) Short Circuit
(4) Drawing Out
(5) Putting In

In these instructions the one giving the treatment is called the *Operator*, and the one being treated is called the *Recipient*.

CORRECTING POLARITY

Obviously the Magnetism in our bodies must be balanced and flowing correctly before we can either be treated or give treatment Magnetically.

The first step in giving a treatment is to correct the recipient's polarity. What exactly is "polarity"? Polarity is the way Magnetism is flowing in the body. Correct polarity is the steady, uninterrupted, flow of life-force from the negative poles of your body to the positive poles of your body. That is, the life-force is entering your body through your negative hand and foot, flowing through your entire system (just as blood flows through your veins), and then flowing out through your positive foot and hand. Perhaps an even more accurate example is your breathing. Your lungs take in fresh air; it is circulated through the body; and then you breathe out the air—now laden with the impurities and toxins collected by its passage through the body. Your body does the same thing with life-force. We can even say that your nervous system "breathes," too. And just as illness and death can result from inadequate breathing or suffocation, so also inadequate or blocked flow of the life-force in your body can result in disease and even death.

Confused Polarity

Polarity can become "confused" as well as weakened or blocked.

By "confused" we mean that the direction of its flow gets altered and switched around in parts of the body. This causes blockage, leaks, or malfunctioning of a body part—just as a motor will begin running backwards if you switch its poles. So a reversed, confused flow of life-force can make a body part "go haywire."

Checking Polarity

The best way to check for confused polarity is to have a person remove their shoes and put their feet up (better if they simply lie down). Then, Draw Out (see page 26) from their positive foot. If the Magnetic flow is good and strong, then their polarity is fine, and they do not need any correction at that time. But if it is weak (maybe even coming in faint spurts) or undetectible, they need their polarity corrected.

Correcting Another's Polarity

I will give the description of Polarity Correction for another person, as it will make the instruction for correcting your own polarity easier to understand.

(1) Have the recipient lie down, relaxed and with hands at the sides and legs slightly separated.

(2) Hold your hands—palm downward, the fingers held straight out and parallel with the ground (the tips pointing in the direction of the recip-

15

ient's head) three to five inches above the recipient's head (see Fig. 6A).

(3) Beginning at the top of the recipient's head, cross and uncross your arms—palms downward toward the recipient—in a side-to-side sweeping motion, moving steadily down to the bottoms of the feet. Keep your hands three to five inches above the recipient's body (see Figs. 6B, 6C and 6D).

(4) This is done the entire length of the recipient's body a total of four times:

(a) Twice with your positive hand closer to the recipient, and your negative hand crossing above it.

(b) Twice with your negative hand closer to the recipient, and your positive hand crossing above it.

(5) Do not move too rapidly toward the recipient's feet. Move down just a hand's breadth at the end of each sidewise sweep.

Correcting Your Own Polarity

(1) Lie down.

(2) Hold your two hands over your head, three to five inches above your body.

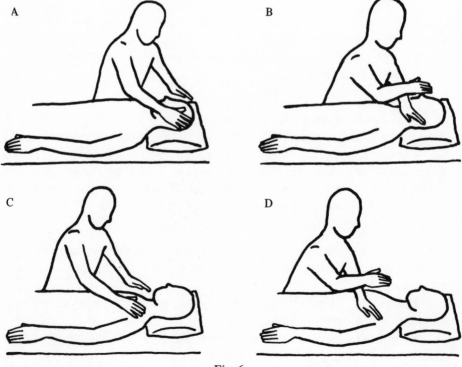

Fig. 6

(3) The fingers of your hands should be pointing toward the top of of your head (see Fig. 7A).

(4) Using the same side-to-side sweep of the hands, as in correcting another's polarity, and moving down toward your feet after each sweep (see Figs. 7B, 7C and 7D), continue until you can no longer keep your hands positioned correctly and yet have your fingers pointing toward your head.

(5) Turn your hands so the fingertips are toward your feet (see Fig. 7E); and continue on (see Fig. 7F) to just beyond your feet. Of course, you will have to sit up in order to move your hands over the lower parts of your body.

(6) Do this four times as outlined in Correcting Another's Polarity, section 4.

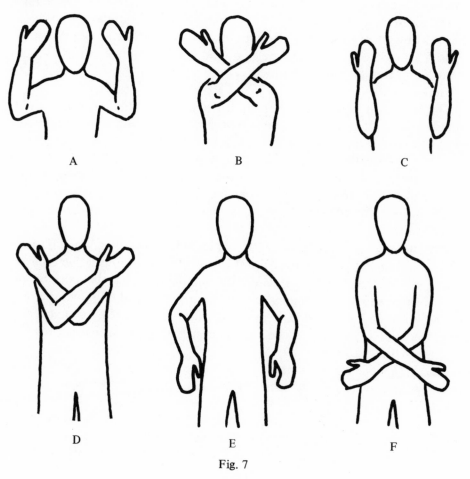

A   B   C

D   E   F

Fig. 7

Now your polarity is corrected.

Do not underestimate the value of this simple Polarity Correction. Confused polarity causes many diseases and mental instability ("nerves"); and this Polarity Correction goes right to the root of the malfunction and corrects it.

BODY SWEEP

Magnetism is not only flowing through and throughout the body, it is also circulating around it in a measurable magnetic field. This is the "aura" we so often hear about. This magnetic field also becomes disturbed or weakened—sometimes negative life-force circulates in the aura before being absorbed by the body and causing disease or lowered vitality. The Body Sweep therefore does two things: it stimulates the healthy flow of Magnetism around the body, balances and regulates that flow, and eliminates negative life-force that might be there. Further, it draws a considerable portion of any negative life-force out of the body, and eliminates it. This is a fundamental healing method, and is of inestimable worth. It is a "must" in every Magnetic treatment.

Here is how:

(1) Have the recipient either sit on a chair or stand (I think that standing is better, myself). Be sure they are standing or sitting with enough room for you to walk around them in a circle.

(2) Stand directly in front of the recipient.

(3) Cup your hands slightly, and bring them up and hold them, *palms down* and thumbs touching, about one inch over the recipient's head. Even closer is all right, but the recipient's body should not be touched in the Body Sweep.

(4) Slowly and smoothly—with hands still cupped and palms held downward—separate your hands and move them down on either side of the recipient's head and neck; along the shoulders; down the sides of his arms (which should be hanging relaxed by his side) and on down the rest of his body and sides of his legs to the floor (see Fig. 8), keeping your hands near the body—no more than one inch away, less, if it is possible to do so without touching it.

Note that the hands are always on opposite sides of the recipient's body, as though his body was a pivot point around which your hands are turning on an axis.

(5) Then, forming your hands into fists, rise up and at the same time flick your fingers outward while shaking your hands also outward with a "snap" away from the recipient's body (see Fig. 8), as though shaking

18

off the negative energy gathered by your hands. Remember: never turn the palms of your hands toward the recipient when doing this. Instead, always keep the hands slightly cupped and palms downward when making the sweeping motions.

(6) Bring your hands back up to above the recipient's head with an outward curving sweeping motion, again cupping them and being sure that the palms are turned downward. (As I said, imagine that your two hands are moving on an axis with the recipient's body as the pivot point.) Thus the hands are always directly opposite to one another with the recipient's body always in between them.

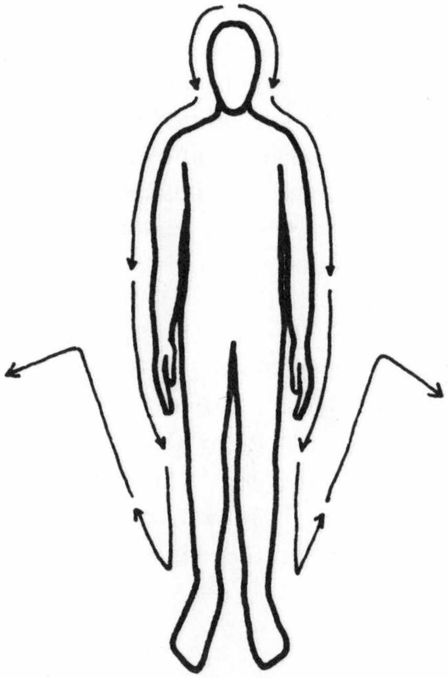

Fig. 8

(7) With this imaginary axis in mind, turn your hands slightly on a left-to-right, clockwise pivot, and again bring them down over the recipient's body in the sweeping motion. This time, however, your right hand will not be at the exact side of the head and body, but rather about a palm's breadth over to the right—more toward the front of the recipient's face. Coming down further, your right hand will be to the right of where it was before, and thus just in front of his left arm and the trunk of his body. Your left hand will be just behind his right shoulder. Again, after you have swept down the whole length of his body, shake your hands out as outlined above.

(8) Return your hands to above the recipient's head—cupped slightly and palms held downward.

(9) This time you move the hands on their imaginary axis a little further in a left-to-right, clockwise circle, and again make a full body sweep. This time your right hand will be descending nearly in front of the center of the recipient's face, and your left hand will be nearly opposite his spine. After completing the sweep to the floor, shake your hands, flicking the fingers, as described, and again return the hands to above his head.

(10) This time when you sweep down, your right hand will be descending right in the center of the recipient's face, just in front of his nose, and your left hand will be passing directly down the line of the spine.

19

(Remember not to touch him.)

(11) In this way, keep moving your hands on the imaginary axis and sweeping down to the floor, until you have circled him completely, and find yourself standing in front of the recipient in your original position.

(12) Repeat the above, entire process at least once—if not twice—more.

This completes the Body Sweep.

For seriously ill persons, you may wish to do the Body Sweep several times in succession.

I find that when working with an average-size adult it takes *twelve* sweeps in this way to circle around the recipient thoroughly (see Fig. 9). And thoroughness counts greatly here. Think of the body as divided into four parts: (1) Left shoulder to center of face; (2) Center of face to right shoulder; (3) Right shoulder to center of back (spine); (4) Center of back to left shoulder. And three sweeps are required to cover each area. Naturally, there will be some overlapping on the head and neck since their circumference is so small. But that is all right.

Four Important Points

Four things are crucial in doing the Body Sweep:

(1) Keep your hands cupped throughout the downward sweep.

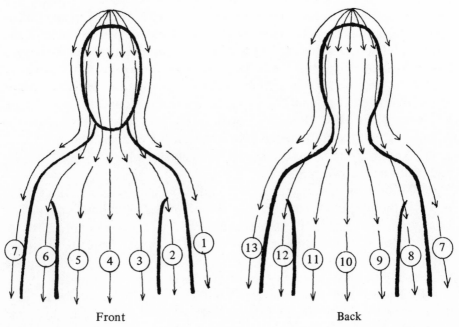

Front   Back

Fig. 9

20

(2) Keep your hands held with palms down throughout the sweep and NEVER turn them toward the recipient.

(3) Form your hands into fists after each sweep and then flick out the fingers away from the recipient, while snapping your hands in a shaking motion (also away from the recipient) when rising up to begin the next sweep.

(4) WASH YOUR HANDS RIGHT AFTER DOING THIS. Wash your hands and forearms in cold water. Running water is best. (If you do not have it at hand, then use a basin of cold water—and swish your hands around in the water vigorously.) Then "squeegie" the water off each hand with the opposite one (see

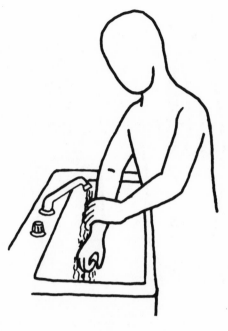

Fig. 10

Fig. 10). And then "squeegie" off each finger individually. If you are using a sink it is also good to touch the metal spigot with all your finger-tips and thumbs. This will also help in drawing off any negative Magnetism you have collected on your hands. *This is always done after any Magnetic work (including Long Distance), no matter how slight,* for it is possible to pick up the recipient's disorders if the negative Magnetism is not eliminated from your hands and body.

SHORT CIRCUIT

The third technique is that which we call the Short Circuit. It consists simply of holding the two hands—palms facing each other (see Fig. 11)—on opposite sides of the body or body part, such as the recipient's leg, arm, or head. The two hands should be positioned so that the fingers are also opposite one another and pointing in the same direction. In Egypt, ancient carvings in the rocks show healers treating patients by placing one hand on the patient's stomach and the other on his back, just opposite the hand in front.

The Short Circuit is usually employed on the head (hands on either side) to treat headaches or effect the pituitary gland (in cases of high or low blood pressure). It can also be used for treating the ears on some

21

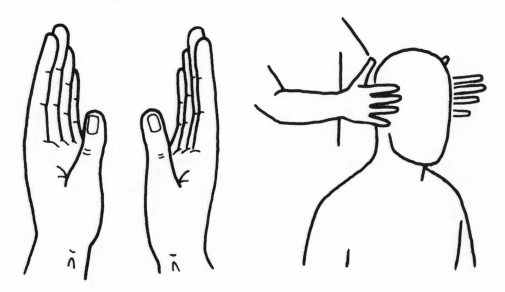

Fig. 11

Fig. 12

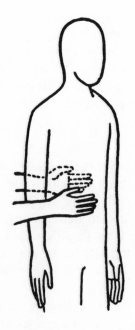

Fig. 13

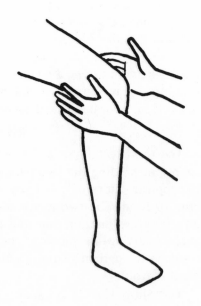

Fig. 14

cases. (See Fig. 12)

Although the Short Circuit can be used to good effect on the internal organs—especially lungs, heart, liver, kidneys, gall bladder, etc. (see Fig. 13)—its particular application is in the treatment of the joints of the body (see Fig. 14) and also the vertebrae of the neck.

Holding the hands on opposite sides of the body part being treated— the palms turned toward each other—keep them there for at least three to five minutes. You do not actually touch the body, but hold your hands away from the body (I prefer about one-and-one-half inches, but for most people the distance is three to six inches—for some it is one foot away.), at whatever distance you feel is the most effective. You can pretty much just go by "feel" in this matter.

When working on a body organ or an area of the body, rather than on the head or joints, your negative hand should be behind and your positive hand in front, so the Magnetism will flow from your negative hand to your positive hand, thereby flowing into the part being treated. THE ONE EXCEPTION IS THE SHORT CIRCUIT ON THE HEART. In that situation, your negative hand should be in front of the heart area and your positive hand in back. This is most important.

You can apply the Short Circuit for as long as ten minutes in one position, but no longer (at one time, that is), unless the problem is gravely serious.

As a rule, you should never work on any spot for more than ten minutes at a time.

In applying the Short Circuit you may need to try a few positions in relation to the joints or vertebrae of the neck. For example, I have found that when using the Short Circuit on a joint it is consistently best to hold the hands on the sides of the joints or neck. But you may find instances where holding the hands in front and behind the joints or neck will be more effective.

The exception to what I have just said, is the Short Circuit on the head. When working on the head, it is essential that we not confuse the recipient's polarity—which we will do if we are not careful. The head is itself a magnet—one side is positive and the other is negative. Therefore the Magnetic flow in a person's head is naturally moving from negative to positive. (All Magnetism flows from negative to positive. It is a "law" of Magnetism.)

If the operator's negative hand is held on the negative side of the recipient's head, and the operator's positive hand is held on the positive side of the recipient's head, the Magnetic flow will be harmonious, for the

Magnetism flowing from the operator's negative hand toward his positive hand will blend with that flowing from the negative side of the recipient's head to the positive side (see Fig. 15). *But* if the operator's negative hand is held at the positive side of the recipient's head, and his positive hand on the negative side of the recipient's head, the flow between the operator's hands will conflict with the natural flow in the recipient's head; and the recipient's polarity will become confused or even reversed! I know this, because such a thing happened to me.

One operator placed his hands incorrectly in relation to the positive and negative sides of my head. Right away I felt much discomfort, but

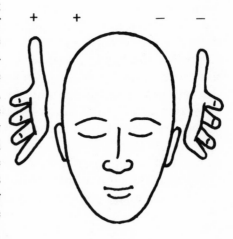

Fig. 15

thought it was just a peculiar reaction on my part. After a while it became unbearable and I demanded that he stop the Short Circuit. Then we realized the cause of the problem. My polarity was corrected again by the operator and the Short Circuit done in the right way. This gave me relief from really terrible discomfort and headache, but a mild, ill-at-ease sensation persisted for a few hours.

So we must beware: *A misapplied Short Circuit is the only way in which we can harm a patient.* And it is no joke. It is my opinion (untested, unproved) that besides physical problems, much mental illness stems from confused polarity. As I say, this is no joke.

All right: how do we avoid misapplying the Short Circuit? The principle is this: ALWAYS hold your negative hand on the negative side of the recipient's head, and your positive hand on the positive side of the recipient's head. In brief: *Match* your polarity with that of the recipient.

Here is another short "rule of thumb": If the recipient has the *same* handedness as you, stand *behind* him to do the Short Circuit (see Fig. 16A). If the recipient has a *different* handedness than you, stand *in front* of him for the Short Circuit (see Fig. 16B).

Now, just what is the nature of a Short Circuit? When you oppose the palms of your hands, you produce a Magnetic flow between them, from the negative hand to the positive hand (see Fig. 17), just as when two poles of a battery are connected or you oppose the positive pole of a magnet with the negative pole of another magnet. And, as I have said, your two hands are positive and negative poles of your body-magnet. So when you oppose your hands to each other on either side of a body part, the resulting Magnetic flow passes through that part, effecting it strongly. Not only does it correct the Magnetism of the body part, it can actually break up deposits in the joints and vertebrae. Later on we will be considering the use of the Short Circuit to actually crumble kidney and gall stones.

The Short Circuit is even used sometimes in hospitals when a mild electric current is passed through the heart of cardiac patients, from back to front, by means of electrical equipment. So the principle of the Short Circuit is known to "regular medicine" as well.

Distance Of The Hands

Here we should consider the matter of how far the hands are held from the body of the recipient—for we do not touch the body itself in Magnetic Therapy. "Magnetism at a certain distance produces a greater effect than when it is applied immediately" (Mesmer). I find that holding my hands only about one-and-a-half inches from the recipient's body is most effec-

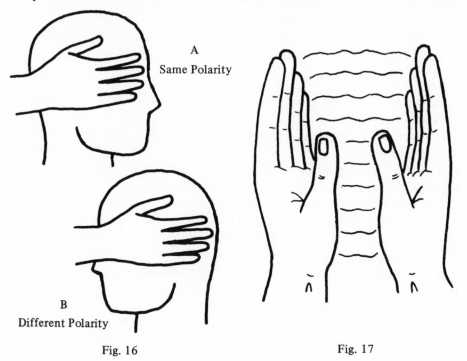

A
Same Polarity

B
Different Polarity

Fig. 16

Fig. 17

tive for *me*, and certainly makes it easier for me to feel the Magnetic flow. But usually people find that three to five inches is more comfortable or "natural feeling" to them. Some even find that they work best if they actually do place their hands on the recipient. But I urge you to try applying Magnetism without actually touching the recipient before you decide definitely you need to place your hands directly on those you treat. This is because the sensitivity of your hands to the Magnetic flow will be hindered by the sensations of clothing texture. Even more important, since you need to be guided by the sensations of heat or electrical flow emanating from the leaks of the recipient's body, you may mistake the recipient's natural body heat for the heat of Magnetic leaks. Also, the recipient sometimes should guide you by *his* sensations of the Magnetism flowing to him from your hands, and if your hands are touching him the warmth he will feel from your hands may interfere with that.

If, however, you find you cannot effectively apply Magnetism except by laying your hands directly on the recipient's body, then go right ahead. But do keep in mind that you will not always be able to rely on either your own or the recipient's sensations of heat-flow. Further, as previously said, the sensation of touching the recipient's clothes may cancel out your feeling of the Magnetic flow from your hands. Although this is not absolutely essential, it is a major factor in helping the operator know when he has worked long enough on a particular spot.

DRAWING OUT

Next we come to the most important technique of Magnetic Therapy: Drawing Out.

Hippocrates wrote: "It has often appeared while I have been soothing my patient that there was a strange property in my hands to pull and draw away from the affected parts aches, and diverse impurities, by laying my hand upon the place." He was referring to Drawing Out.

This method has a fourfold benefit: (1) It increases the flow of life-force into the body; (2) it removes blockages of the life-force; (3) it causes diseased or damaged parts of the body to become "saturated" with life-force and thus stimulates the healing power of the body; (4) it removes negative life-force that may have accumulated in a particular area of the body. This fourth point is perhaps the most important, especially in dealing with disease caused by poisons in the organs or tissues. It is also of prime importance in treating cysts and tumors. Except for the few types of problems where the Short Circuit or Putting In is of most benefit, the method of Drawing Out is to be used in treating all complaints. This one method can be used in *all* situations, but there are times when the others will produce a quicker result.

The method of Drawing Out is this:

(1) Place your negative hand—open with the palm toward the recipient's body—over the area of the body where there is pain or disease: not touching the body, but above it at the distance you have found best for you.

(2) Hold your positive hand out and down, open with the palm turned downward and parallel to the ground (see Fig. 18).

You will no doubt feel heat, stinging, or tingling in the palm of both hands. By holding your hands in this way you make your body into a great, drawing magnet. The life-force begins flowing from the recipient's "trouble spot," through your negative hand and arm, and out through your positive arm and hand. Thus Drawing Out accomplishes all the four effects listed at the beginning of this section. And right away.

At this point three questions arise:

(1) If you draw life-force out of the recipient's body, won't the recipient's body become depleted of life-force?

Answer: No. Just the opposite. The human body is set up to be continually drawing life-force into itself and throwing it off. This is done

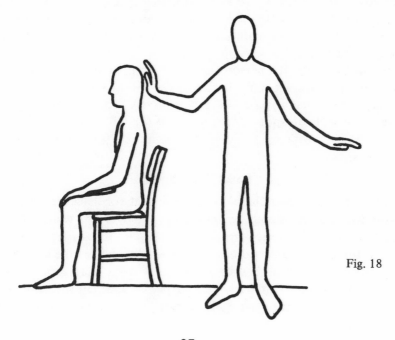

Fig. 18

27

by means of the poles of the body-magnet. When the life-force becomes blocked the body's drawing power is weakened. But if you begin drawing from any spot of the body, the impeded clogged life-force is freed, begins to flow vigorously, and automatically the influx of life-force is increased. Thus, even though you may be working on only one spot, the entire body becomes revitalized. Many times, as you are Drawing Out, sensitive recipients will feel tingling or warmth in their negative hands and feet as the flow of life-force into their bodies is stimulated.

(2) If you draw negative life-force from ill recipients through your own body, will you then become ill?

Answer: There is a definite possibility that if negative life-force becomes lodged in your body, you may become ill yourself. This can be avoided by three things: (a) When you are finished Drawing Out, slowly move your negative hand away from the recipient's body, and raise it in the position for Putting In (see page 31). Hold this position for about thirty seconds. By doing this you will draw pure life-force into yourself and any negative life-force between the two poles of your hands will flow right on out of your positive hand—which should still be held down and out, away from the recipient. (b) To further insure getting rid of all negative life-force, you must unfailingly wash your hands carefully as has been described before in the section on the Body Sweep. (c) You must keep your own body in good health. Good health creates a positive Magnetism in the body that can counteract and neutralize negative Magnetism. But health must be maintained! This is why I have included a section on Staying Healthy.

(3) How long should a person Draw Out from a recipient?

Answer: The average time is five to ten minutes on one spot (though you may treat many spots in a treatment). The maximum time for treatment of a single spot is ten minutes. (*Why* will be discussed later.) Of course, you can work on many spots—the limit is just on the time on any particular spot.

Small "Hot Spots"

Often, when Drawing Out you will feel heat (or "electricity") emanating from the recipient's body to your palm. Then, after a while—sometimes quickly or sometimes only after several minutes—the sensation of heat or electrical tingling in your palm ceases. When this occurs the leak is sealed, the negative Magnetism has been removed from that area. Then you should stop Drawing Out from that particular spot. In subsequent treatments, though, test the spot again, and if you feel heat, then Draw Out

28

again.

(4) What if a recipient has pain in a spot and you feel no heat or electrical tingling there?

Answer: Chances are the pain is symptomatic of a problem in another area. But go ahead and Draw Out from the place of pain for five to ten minutes (or until the pain stops). Since that spot is paining, it is somehow connected with the actual trouble spot, and Drawing Out from it will effect the real problem area. Once, for two days I had a terrible sinus headache—or so I thought. The morning of the second day I had had enough of it, so I asked one of our Monastery residents to do Magnetic for me, and Draw Out from my aching sinuses. (I was so long in getting treated because I had not much experience with Magnetism then, and still could hardly believe its effectiveness.) He began Drawing Out, and immediately I had the peculiar sensation of a magnetic "cord" running down to my stomach and drawing it upward. It felt just as though a magnet were pulling on it. So I told him to quit Drawing Out from my head and instead Draw Out from my stomach area. He did so for only a few minutes, and that was the end of the headache! But if I had not been sensitive like that, working on my head area would still have helped— indeed, it was the effecting of the stomach that I was feeling in that pulling sensation.

(5) Are there situations when Drawing Out should not be done?

Answer: Yes! NEVER Draw Out from the heart or the solar plexus. Only Put In (to be discussed next) to these body parts. When there is a problem with the heart, and you feel that Drawing Out is called for, then Draw Out from the *back*—just opposite the heart.

Using Your Hands As Sensors

Drawing Out has another function besides simple treatment. Through the Drawing Out positioning of your hands, you can use your negative hand as a "sensor" to search out trouble spots and, after treating them, to tell when the Magnetism is corrected.

Nearly all—if not all—disease or physical malfunctions emanate a Magnetic field, or flow, that is picked up by the palm as heat or electrical tingling in Drawing Out. When that Magnetism enters your negative palm as it is being drawn out, the palm feels this as heat, tingling, stinging, etc. Often the same sensation is felt by the palm of your positive hand as it leaves your body. Whenever such sensations are picked up by your palm, stay on that spot and Draw Out. When the sensation stops (not just lessens), move the palm over the nearby area—often you will encounter milder or more intense "hot spots." Draw Out from these, too. Sometimes you may feel heat in your fingertips, but not the palm: *only pay attention to the palm*. I am saying "palm," but frequently people feel heat not in the middle of the palm (I do) but at the base of the palm, the "heel" of the hand. That is also correct and reliable.

Anyhow, use your negative palm and its sensations to determine how long to Draw Out. Sometimes you will pass over a "hot spot," pause, and it will "fade" in a matter of seconds. Why? Because it is simply an emanation from a nerve plexus connected with a troubled area. Several times I have checked the positions of these "hot flashes" on an Acupuncture chart and found that they corresponded to Acupuncture points.

But what if the heat, tingling, or stinging does *not* stop after ten minutes of Drawing Out? You should stop Drawing Out on that particular spot anyway, and come back to it in the next treatment. This is of prime importance, as will be explained later in the section on Reactions.

One thing you may encounter: while Drawing Out, the sensation of heat suddenly turns to *cold*. This means the polarity has changed, the "leak" has sealed, and you need no longer continue working on that spot. This is very rare, but you may come across it in your work with Magnetism.

Two Hints On Increasing
The Efficiency of Drawing Out

(1) Since you are making your body into a magnet it will definitely assume a relationship with the greater magnet of the earth. We have found that the effectiveness of Drawing Out is markedly increased if the fingers of your positive hand (which is being held down and parallel with the floor, the palm facing downward) are pointing toward the *South* (see Fig. 19). This was discovered by Mesmer, who wrote: "If the current of the Magnetism concurs in its direction with the general current,

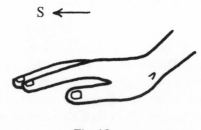

Fig. 19

or with the Magnetic current of the earth, the general result is an increase of intensity of all these currents."

(2) As I will be discussing later, you do not visualize or affirm that the Magnetism is flowing through you. Rather, you should be calm, even detached, and let the natural flow of the Magnetism take place. But it *has*

been found that if you make yourself very aware of—intently "feel"—the sensations of your two palms (especially the positive one), the Magnetic flow will increase. Be sure that you are just being aware of the palms, *not* "directing" the Magnetic flow.

I hope you will read over this section on Drawing Out several times— there are so many important points in it that are essential to correct, effective practice.

PUTTING IN

Drawing Out is the main technique of Magnetic Therapy. However, you may find some instances where Drawing Out makes the recipient (or even you) very uncomfortable, perhaps even greatly increasing pain in an area. At such a time you may find that Putting In will be more comfortable for the recipient or you. Also, if on some occasion your own vitality is somewhat lowered and you are not too sure that your body could handle any absorption of negative energy from a recipient, you might want to use Putting In. It is, however, my experience that Putting In is not as effective as Drawing Out, as a rule. Once, though, I found that one recipient's cracked rib responded best to Putting In.

The method of Putting In is this:

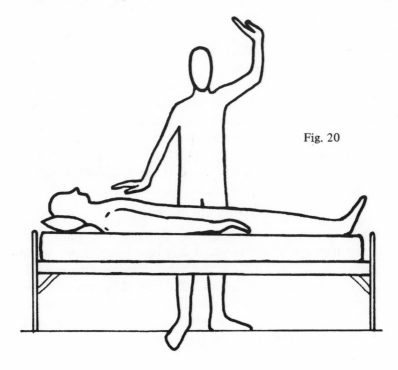

Fig. 20

(1) Place your positive hand over the part of the recipient's body to be treated.

(2) Raise your negative hand over your head, with the palm facing directly upward and your fingers spread and curved as though you are holding a ball in your hand (see Fig. 20).

(3) Just keep that position as long as you wish to be working on the recipient.

In a book on Egyptian antiquities by Montfaucon, a painting is described in which healers are treating a sick person by holding their hands in the Putting In positions. Until the discovery of Magnetic Therapy, such pictures were a great mystery to scholars.

A Hint To Increase Effectiveness

As in Drawing Out, it helps to orient yourself with the Magnetism of the earth. We have found that if your negative hand is held with the heel of your hand toward the *North*—as though your curved fingers were poised to catch a ball thrown from the North—it increases the Magnetic flow considerably (see Fig. 21).

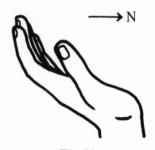

Fig. 21

As in Drawing Out, if your positive hand feels a sensation of cold, it means that the leak in the recipient's body is sealed, and you need no longer work on that particular spot in that treatment. (This does *not* mean you should not work on it in future treatments.) Sometimes you may feel your palms being repelled—pushed away from the recipient—as though a balloon is being squashed between your hand and the recipient's body. That, too, indicates that the leak is sealed, and no more Magnetism is entering the recipient's body at that particular spot.

Clearing The Room

After every treatment with Magnetic Therapy, the room should be cleared of any negative Magnetism that may have been drawn out into the air. To do this, open the windows and have a fan blowing out. It is also very good to burn incense in the room. Sandalwood incense is the absolute best, but frankincense mixed with a little Benzoin (Sumatra) is excellent. Be sure you do not have negative Magnetism circulating around to be absorbed by you or others who enter the room.

WHAT YOU DO NOT DO

You do not heal. This has already been considered.

You do not diagnose. This is the province of qualified medical practitioners. Anyway, we are simply working on the Magnetism of the body—not on disease or even the body itself—so what need do we have to diagnose? We are not practicing medicine, we are simply balancing the Magnetism of the body and facilitating its natural curative property.

You do not "direct" the Magnetic energy. The simple placement of your hands is sufficient. In this way you ensure that the Magnetic flow is *natural*, therefore the most effective.

You do not "suggest," "affirm," or visualize in any way. If you do, you limit and hinder the flow of Magnetism, which is a force much greater and more subtle than mere mental energy. To attempt mental manipulation of this fundamental force is to actually decrease its effectiveness. The temptation to "play healer" must be resisted, both for your own sake and that of the recipient. The great Magnetic therapist, F.W. Sears, wrote: "Every life is a vital center through which the All-Health energy of the universe is pouring all the time, when it is not obstructed by our own personal thought currents. I never use my personal energy. There is where many healers make a big mistake. They have a consciousness that it is their personal force, their personal self, their personal power that is healing the patient. The result is they give of themselves, and while it is true they effect some cures, such cures are at the expense of their own vitality. This occurs only when we use a personal force, for the law of the personal plane of consciousness is destructive. So in giving treatments we should never live in the consciousness that it is our personal force, that it is we who are doing it. Live in the consciousness that we are the connecting link through which the All-Health energy of the universe is pouring, just as the pipe which conducts the water from the source of supply is the connecting link between the source and the faucet."

3

THERAPY ROUTINES

First, be sure that you are yourself in good health! Never, never work on anyone else when you are not in good shape. Otherwise you will pass on some of your illness (no matter how minor) to them, and in your weakened resistance will absorb their problems. In this way you will just be playing a "musical chairs" game with illness. Don't—for your sake and that of the recipient.

Although in a pinch we can work on just trouble spots, it is always best to give a full treatment, which is as follows.

(1) First, see that neither you nor the recipient are wearing any metal or material (silk, wool, or leather) which can impede the Magnetic flow. Also, that neither you nor the recipient are touching metal in any way.

(2) Check the recipient's polarity (see page 15). If it needs correction, do so. (Your own polarity should have already been corrected.)

(3) Twice (at least) do the Body Sweep on the recipient.

(4) Wherever the recipient has a problem or pain, Draw Out at those spots until the sensation of heat or electricity (if any) subsides. If the sensations do not cease, then keep Drawing Out until you have Drawn Out for ten minutes—no more—on each spot.

(Another good General Routine is to search all over the recipient's head area, using your negative hand as a sensor while Drawing Out. Then do the same search down the spine, clear to the base. When all "hot spots" are eliminated from the head and spine, you can be pretty sure that the rest of the body is all right, since all body parts are connected to the head and spine.)

(5) WASH YOUR HANDS. *Always* wash your hands.

Intensive Treatment Routine

Normally the preceding five steps are enough for a treatment. But if the recipient is in poor health, it may be good to give a more intensive treatment. To do that, besides what is outlined in the four steps above, also make a thorough search of the recipient's body, holding your hands in the Drawing Out position and carefully moving your negative hand—at a slight distance—over the recipient's entire body: both front and back—using your negative hand as a "sensor" to pick up the sensations of heat or electrical flow which indicate leaks or problems in the body. Wherever you find heat or electrical tingling, Draw Out from that spot (or Put In or apply the Short Circuit, if that seems best) until the sensations stop or ten minutes have passed. Then move on.

Three further questions need to be considered in this section:

(1) *How many treatments should a person have?* A person with a specific problem should be treated until the problem is removed; and then at least three more treatments should be given to make sure the problem is truly removed and not just alleviated or in abeyance.

"Do not be deceived with the idea that the relief which follows a Magnetic treatment is permanent—that is to say, that a chemical change has taken place and that the symptom is permanently cured because it has disappeared. The relief which follows a Magnetic treatment is due to the fact that artificial stimulus has been supplied to the nerve centers. They are able to do their work much more effectively than they did before, but they are doing this work with a force other than their own. After a while, in the course of time, it will be discovered that the special stimulus has been exhausted, consequently the patient will be in the same condition as before. The Magnetic treatments, therefore, must be continued for some time after the patient is apparently cured, until the defect has been removed, and the patient has had a chance to accumulate the necessary amount of energy unto the successful performance of the work.

"In a word, a permanent cure is one thing; the relief of disease symptoms by Magnetic treatment is quite another" (Dr. A.S. Raleigh).

(2) *Can you "overload" the recipient with Magnetism?* No, because when the amount of Magnetism in the recipient is brought up to the right level, no more will be absorbed by him. As mentioned before, you may even feel "cold" in your palm, or have the sensation that your hand is being repelled from the surface of his body, much like the feeling of having a balloon squashing between his body and your hand. This is one of the advantages of Magnetic Therapy. A person can take too much of a certain kind of medicine—or even the wrong kind of medicine. But in Magnetic Therapy this cannot happen. Actually, one of the criteria of health is that exteriorly applied Magnetism ceases to effect the recipient. When this happens, they are well. Magnetism is a universal force that operates by precise laws of need and supply. Not one unit is wasted. The moment a recipient needs no more Magnetism, in that moment Magnetism ceases to flow to him from the operator. This does not mean that no

further therapy is needed, but *at that moment* the maximum has been accomplished.

Even a person without any specific problem would do well to have a full Magnetic treatment periodically. In our Monastery each member has a Body Sweep and "search" over the head and spine done once a week as a matter of routine.

(3) *How often should a person be treated?* You should not treat a recipient within less than seventy-two hours after the previous treatment—unless some *new* problem arises that requires attention. This is because Magnetic Therapy, simple though it may be, affects the body profoundly, producing radical and subtle changes. Therefore enough time must be given for the recipient's body to adjust before further treatment. For this reason, no one should have their eyes tested or have a physical examination (unless ill) within seventy-two hours after a Magnetic treatment, because the reactions and adjustments the body undergoes might cause an incorrect result in the test. It is actually a very good thing for the recipient to lie down and sleep for some time after the therapy, as the body is adjusting itself initially.

REACTIONS

Considering the foregoing, this may be the most appropriate place to discuss *reactions*. Mesmer, in his Maxims regarding this type of therapy, wrote: "We can also understand that the application of Magnetism frequently increases the suffering. (212) It is through the application of Magnetism that the symptoms cease. (214) Furthermore, it is also through Magnetism that the efforts of Nature against the causes of disease are increased, and consequently the critical symptoms are increased. (215)"

Magnetic Therapy is not a surface treatment: it deals with the fundamental element of our physical existence: life-force, itself. So when we undergo Magnetic treatment a profound change occurs. The effect is *natural,* but so are volcanic eruptions and tornadoes! One Magnetic treatment can so revitalize the body that many toxins are expelled by the newly-awakened system. As a result a recipient may even feel worse than he did before the treatment. This is not the rule, but it does happen. For this reason we do not work on a spot more than ten minutes at one time nor before seventy-two hours have elapsed between treatments. The old Magnetic "healers" of the past placed much emphasis upon the *crisis*—a violent reaction that they claimed was essential to recovery of health.

Jerome Eden in *Animal Magnetism and the Life Energy* discusses the phenomenon of crisis/reactions thus: "Without going into the details of

36

this aberration, which is almost general and all but restricted to living matter, it is easy to conceive, according to a general law, that an impulse toward movement is always met by a resisting effort, and that the impulse toward movement must be adjusted so that it overcomes the resisting effort. This effort is called *crisis*, and all the effects which result directly from this crisis are called *critical symptoms*. They are the true means of recovery, or what constitutes *the natural cure*; whereas the effects stemming from the resistance to this natural effort are called *symptomatic symptoms*. These produce what is called the *illness*. . . .

"Hippocrates seems to have been the first and perhaps the only one who grasped the phenomena of crises in critical diseases. He recognized that the different symptoms were only modifications of the efforts which nature makes against diseases. After him, however, whenever men observed the same symptoms in chronic illnesses, far removed from their initial causes, and without the fever attendant upon critical diseases, they isolated these symptoms, fabricated many 'diseases,' and characterized each *with a different name*."

It is true that our systems must be stirred up to heal themselves, but obviously these old-timers over-treated at each session and definitely too frequently—usually daily. Mesmer's patients frequently went into convulsions! However, not one person ever suffered ill effects in the long run. But caution should be our watchword. We should not be fearful, but we should be scrupulously careful. If we do not work on a spot more than ten minutes, and do not work on a recipient less than seventy-two hours between sessions, we should not have difficulties with severe reactions. But reactions there will be to some extent, though mostly mild—even to the point of going unnoticed. We should, though, be vigilant, keeping these things in mind. My warning not to overtreat or work on someone at too short intervals is based on sober realities.

Exceptions?

Are there any exceptions to the ten-minutes-seventy-two-hours-apart rule? Almost none. As I said before, if the case is very serious, and a reaction would not be as bad as the present state of the problem, you might *cautiously* work a little more or a little more frequently. Some types of problems actually require a longer working time, such as kidney stones (to be discussed in the next chapter). But here, especially, "discretion is the better part of valor." While I am writing this, I have an ache in one body part as a reaction to Magnetic treatment given several hours ago. From past experience I know that this is the prelude to complete

37

relief of the problem I was treated for. But I am also quite aware of what terrible pain I would be in if I had been worked on for a longer period of time or in less than seventy-two hours. I know of one case where a form of Magnetic treatment (*not* according to the methods outlined in this book) was given for *several hours daily* to a college instructor who had bursitis that he wanted cleared up before a brief vacation period was over and he would have to return to teaching. The result was that he had to be hospitalized and operated upon by a specialist, since the treatment had actually adversely affected even the marrow of the bones, which had to be removed by splitting open those bones. Magnetism is a life-saver and a life-preserver, but you can injure yourself by "overdosing" on anything—even oxygen. By adhering to the rules regarding length and frequency of treatment, only benefit will result from your practice.

Increased Sensitivity To Medicine

Another type of reaction is increased responsiveness to medication. Therefore the recipient who is taking medication of any kind—including herbal or "natural" remedies—should watch carefully to see that he is not overdosing as a consequence of increased sensitivity resulting from the Magnetic Therapy. A Magnetic therapist gave the following account at the beginning of this century that is sobering indeed: "In another case which had been under the care of a physician for six months, medicine failed to reach the vital forces, and a magnetizer was called in. After repeating his treatment for a few times, the condition of the patient was materially changed for the better—the surface from a deathly cold became suffused with a pleasant warm glow, soon followed by perspiration. The attendant thought that one of the powders which had been given by direction of the physician, when in a cold inactive state, might aid in inducing sleep. The circulation being so much more active and life-like after Magnetic treatment than before, the medicine had more effect; and after taking the morphine powder, he slept to wake no more in the body. This shows that medicine is at times inoperative, as in this case, when the system is in a cold, inactive state; but after the stimulus of Magnetic treatment it has its usual effect."

Those who take medication such as insulin should be seriously warned about this aspect of Magnetic Therapy.

Further, we can see that since Magnetism so assists the action of medicine, those who are going to "regular doctors" can benefit from this therapy.

38

KIDNEY STONES AND GALLSTONES

Although I have said that we work on the Magnetism of the body, and not on diseases or specific problems, we naturally are going to encounter situations where a qualified doctor has diagnosed the problem for the recipient. One of the most amazing benefits Magnetic Therapy can impart is in the alleviation of Kidney Stones and Gallstones. Just as Magnetism can break up and disperse deposits in joints (through the Short Circuit), so also it can dissolve these stones. The process is not simple, and can take some hours. Here it is:

Kidney Stones

(1) Place your hands so as to be doing a Short Circuit on the affected kidney. *In this method, you actually place your hands on the recipient's body*. As we usually place the positive hand in front and the negative hand in back when working on other organs, so also in the case of stones we place our positive hand in front and the negative hand in back (see Fig. 22A). In this way the Magnetic current passes through the kidney toward the front of the body. Keep your hands in the Short Circuit position until the recipient feels that the stones have passed out of the kidney into the ureter, under your positive hand. He may have a sensation of the pain moving forward to your positive hand, or he may have the feeling of "worms crawling" in the direction of your hand.

(2) When the recipient feels that the stone(s) has passed into the ureter, then place your negative hand over the spot where your positive hand had been, and place your positive hand over the recipient's bladder (see Fig. 22B).

(3) When the discomfort or "crawling" which the recipient will feel between your two hands has stopped, move your negative hand to the spot over the bladder where your positive hand had been. Then place the index finger and middle finger of your positive hand on the recipient's pubic bone—the fingertips pointing toward the recipient's head (see Fig. 22C). If you apply light pressure, you should be able to feel two small indentations for the tips of the fingers to fit into.

(4) When the recipient feels the urge to urinate, take your hands away *slowly*, so he can use the toilet. You might want the recipient to urinate into a special container so you can see if particles of the stone have actually been passed. (Frequently the stones are so thoroughly dissolved by the Magnetism that no particles large enough to be seen remain.)

Notice that in this method you stay on the spot much longer than the normal ten minutes—in fact, you stay as long as an hour or more, if need

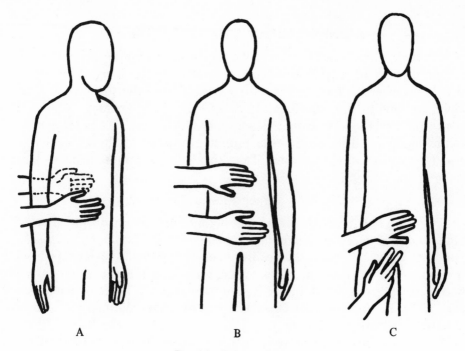

A   B   C

Fig. 22 - Kidney Stones

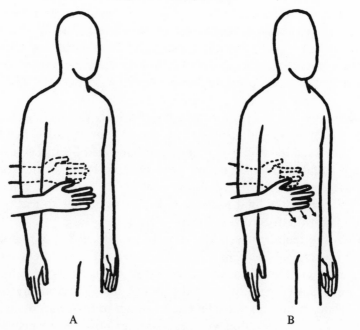

A   B

Fig. 23 - Gallstones

40

be.

Obviously, the above method should not be used on a person under-going a kidney stone attack. Then it is too late, and the sufferer should be taken to a hospital or doctor's office immediately. If, of course, you were miles from any medical facility, it would be good to apply the Short Circuit while on the way to the doctor or hospital, as this could greatly alleviate the pain.

Gallstones

For Gallstones, the process is similar, though not so complex.

(1) Do a Short Circuit on the gall bladder as outlined in the routine for Kidney Stones (see Fig. 23A). Be sure your negative hand is *behind* the recipient's body and your positive hand *in front*. Here, too, you actually touch the recipient's body.

(2) Hold the Short Circuit until the recipient feels through discomfort or a "crawling" sensation that the stones have passed out—or are passing out—into the bile duct.

(3) Then, with your negative hand still held as before, behind the back of the recipient, begin stroking with your positive hand downward toward the duodenum (see Fig. 23B).

(4) After the stones have gone into the duodenum, you need bother no more, as they will from there on be eliminated through the intestines.

The same remarks made in reference to the crumbling and passing of kidney stones given above applies to this method.

Sciatica

(a) Do a Short Circuit, by placing your hands at the sides of the recipient (BE SURE your negative hand is on the recipient's negative side and your positive hand on the positive side), about two inches toward the back, where the muscles form an indentation above the hip joint.

(b) Draw Out over the Sciatic Nerve at the hip joint. Five minutes on each side.

(c) Draw Out from the base of the spine.

Constipation

Do a Short Circuit on the bowels (negative hand in back). Move around to various places, and the recipient should actually feel a "breaking up" sensation. Basically, do as is outlined in the section on Kidney and Gall

41

Stones, even to placing the negative hand above and the positive hand at the base of the spine, near the anus. Be sure a toilet is available!

Headaches

Most headaches can be removed with the Short Circuit. You may need to move around a little bit to find the "hot spots." If the Short Circuit does not give complete relief, then search the head and Draw Out. Migraine headaches can be greatly relieved—and in some cases completely eliminated—in this way, especially if Magnetic is applied from the very beginning of the attack, and again two or three more times that day. No time limit need be observed in working with migraine. Sinus headaches can really be helped with Drawing Out over the sinus cavities.

Joint Problems

Pain, stiffness, and swelling in the joints can be worked on with the Short Circuit. Side to side seems best, but no reason why you shouldn't experiment.

Teeth

Magnetism is no substitute for a good dentist, but we have experienced that tooth pain and especially infection can be helped by Drawing Out. Naturally, cavities and structural problems cannot be cleared up with Magnetism.

Broken Bones

To speed the healing of broken bones, after they are set, apply the Short Circuit especially, but Drawing Out should be tried as well. Even Putting In. See how the recipient feels.

Spine and Coccyx Problems

For bone-related problems, it has been found that Drawing Out greatly helps in actual readjustment of bones (vertebrae). When the problem is muscle spasm (usually bone and muscle problems go together), Putting In seems to work the best to relax the muscles. Use Magnetism to get some relief for these problems, but search out a *good* (adjustment-oriented, drug-avoiding) *Osteopath* for treatment. Some call themselves Osteopaths, but are pill-and-needle pushers out of laziness and incompetence. Select with caution and care (call them on the phone and ask them direct).

Low Vitality

In cases of low vitality—general debility—the Body Sweep and Putting In at the solar plexus (pit of stomach) will be found to help a great deal.

A Further Suggestion

In some recipients it has been found to be more effective if the operator usually Puts In on any spot on the negative side of their body, and Draws Out from places on the positive side of their body. Experiment alone will tell which is best for each individual.

Another Idea to Try

In our experiments with Magnetism, we have observed that the Magnetic flow is markedly enhanced if the *recipient* who is being treated lying down turns his hands up at right angles to his body so both his palms and the soles of his feet are "facing" in the same way (see Fig. 24). This is not essential but it does help. We have tried having the operator close his eyes and simply pick up the "feel" of the Magnetic flow, and in one hundred percent of the tests the operator would always be able to tell when the recipient had "lifted his flippers." Try it for yourself.

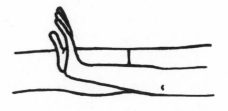

Fig. 24

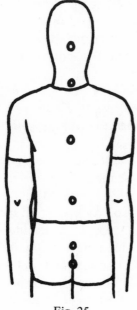

Fig. 25

Spinal Search

Since the body's functions are controlled by nerve centers in the spine, you can also benefit a recipient greatly by searching the spine—from bottom to top—and either Drawing Out or Putting In at each place. Drawing Out is good for malfunction or blockage, and Putting In is best if the problem is a low level of vitality. Fig. 25 shows the main nerve centers (which correspond to the "chakras" of Yoga), but do not confine yourself to them only. In between are also lesser, but vital, nerve centers. These main ones are always worked on in the Spinal Search, however.

43

You Can Treat Yourself

Definitely, you can apply the various methods outlined in this book to help yourself. I believe that it is better to have someone else work on you, but when that is not possible, then apply what you have learned. The Body Sweep cannot be done on yourself to any degree, but certainly Drawing Out, Putting In, and the Short Circuit can be applied by a person on himself.

Team Treatment

There may be a time when you will want to work on a person with increased magnetic force, especially if the recipient really needs rapid assistance (but don't forget about reactions!). To boost your own Magnetism you can have another person help you in working. Here are the ways:

(1) In the techniques of Drawing Out and Putting In, you will find your work greatly facilitated if you have a second operator holding on to the feet (shoes removed, of course) of the recipient. Be sure that the second operator does not confuse the recipient's polarity. The rule is: The second operator holds the *negative* foot of the recipient with his *positive* hand; and the *positive* foot of the recipient with his *negative* hand. This increases the Magnetic flow in the recipient, and itself can clear up many problems. The effect will be as when two magnets become locked together.

Although I speak of the second operator holding the recipient's feet, it is not necessary for him to actually hold them (though I prefer it, myself). The second operator can hold his hands two or three inches away from the bottoms of the recipient's feet (see Fig. 26 A and B), and it will work just fine. Whatever you are most comfortable with.

Here I should mention a rule in Magnetic Therapy that I have not found a place to put in elsewhere: *Never should the recipient's arms or legs be crossed during a treatment; nor should the operator ever cross his arms or legs during a treatment.*

So the immediate question is: If the above is so, how then can a right-handed person hold on to the feet of a left-hander, or vice-versa? The answer is that he will have to stand or sit with his back to the recipient and reach his hands behind himself to do so. Awkward, indeed, but necessary. Of course, if the recipient is lying down, at some time—either when he is lying on his back or is lying on his stomach—this will have to be done, no matter what handedness the second operator and recipient may be. But for working frontwise, the simple rule is: *Face those of your same handedness; turn your back on those of different handedness* (see Fig. 26 A and B). This rule applies when you and the recipient are facing

44

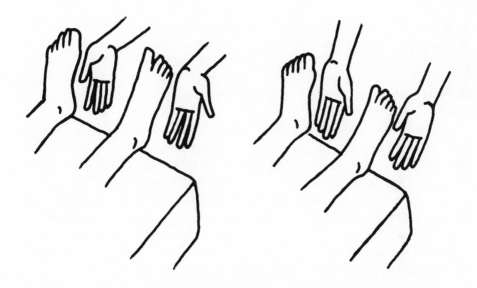

A - Same Handedness

B - Different Handedness

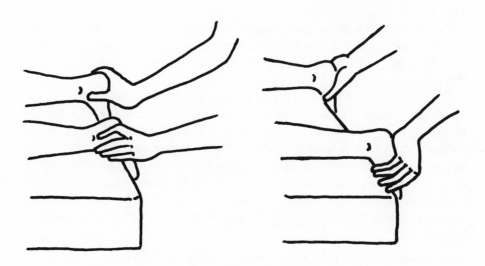

C - Different Handedness

D - Same Handedness

Fig. 26

45

each other, or when the recipient is lying on his back (when you are the second operator and needing to hold his feet). *If, however, the recipient is lying on his stomach, the rule is reversed:* if he has the same handedness as you, then you must turn your back and reach behind you. But if he has a different handedness, then you face him and easily grasp onto his feet (see Fig. 26 C and D).

(2) In doing a Short Circuit, the second operator should stand behind you, placing his hands on your shoulders next to your arms, *if he is of the same handedness as you* (see Fig. 27). If of different handedness, he will have to stand with his back to you, reaching behind him. This cannot practically be done if you are standing, but if you sit down to work on the recipient then it can be done. Personally, I would forget it in this second case and have the second operator hold onto the recipient's feet instead.

One thing that might be done is for the second operator to hold his hands near—not touching—your hands as you do the Short Circuit (see Fig. 28). Be sure his negative hand is held over your negative hand, and his positive hand over your positive hand.

(3) In Putting In, the second operator raises his negative hand as you are doing, but he places his positive hand on your negative shoulder (see Fig. 29).

(4) In Drawing Out, the "tandem" methods outlined above for the Short Circuit and Putting In do not seem to have any value. Having a second operator hold the recipient's feet is however of marked effect in Drawing Out.

In all of these I have simply outlined the participation of a second operator. But there is no reason why there should not be a third, a fourth, or even twenty! I would advise caution, lest you "overload" the recipient with so much high-voltage Magnetism, but in some cases—especially severe ones—it may be the solution. Some of the pioneers in Magnetic therapy, in the eighteenth century, occasionally had every person in the household assist them in this way. But always be sure that the polarities do not get mixed and confused—especially if the people involved are of differing handedness.

LONG DISTANCE TREATMENT

Magnetism is not just universal—it is *unitary*. On the level of this basic life-force there are no divisions, just as an ocean is a unified body. Therefore space is no barrier in dealing with it. *Odd as it may seem, you can treat people from a distance.* My first experience with Magnetism was that of doing a long distance treatment. In that case it was only the distance

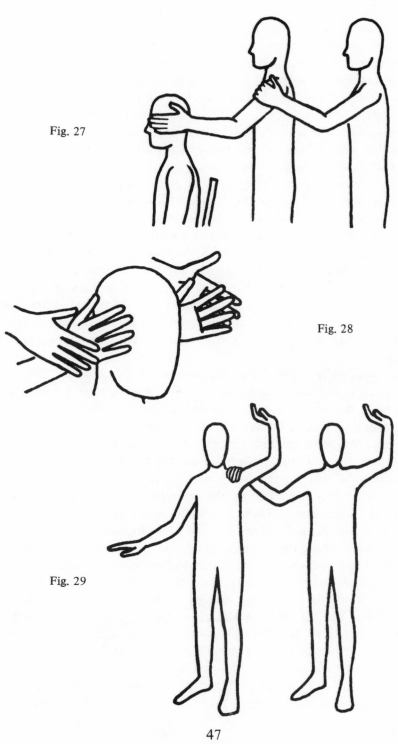

Fig. 27

Fig. 28

Fig. 29

from one room to another. But I understood that if I could do it from a few yards' distance, I could do it from twelve thousand miles away. I was a believer! and since then have proved it to be so.

"The analogy between Absent Treatment and Wireless Telegraphy is almost perfect. If you assume that the Hertzian waves transmitted in wireless telegraphy represent the Healing Magnetism employed in Absent Treatment, then the analogy will be perfect, the ether in either case being the plastic medium between the two instruments, the vibration being the same, that is, as it passes through this plastic medium exercising a corresponding influence upon the organism of the patient.

"Absent Treatment is, therefore, not a figment of the imagination, not an illusion, not a mystical vagary, but is an application of known laws of physics to the healing of the body at a distance from the healer, its laws being the same as any other methods of healing" (Dr. A.S. Raleigh).

Rev. F.W. Sprague, one of the early and most successful of American Magnetic therapists, wrote in the same vein: "The nervous organism acts similar to a wireless telegraphic plant sending out these vital healing forces through the psychic ether and it acts upon that ether through the law of vibration similar to the action of Marconi's electric waves upon the atmosphere."

More technically, Mesmer, in his *Memoir of 1799*, said: "Thus, if a movement of the subtle substance is provoked within a body, there immediately occurs a similar movement in another sensitive to receiving it, whatever the distance between the two persons."

Magnetic therapists are not the only ones who affirm the reality of long distance treatment. Camille Flammarion, the French astronomer, wrote: "The action of one human being upon another, from a distance, is a scientific fact; it is as certain as the existence of Paris, of Napoleon, of Oxygen, or of Sirius. . . . There can be no doubt that our psychical form creates a movement, and the reverse may be analogous to what takes place on a telephone, where the receptive plate, which is identical with the plate at the other end, reconstructs the sonorous movement transmitted, not by means of sound, but by electricity. But these are only comparisons."

Bill Schul, in his book *The Psychic Frontiers of Medicine*, reports: "Several years ago Dr. Robert Miller, an Atlanta chemical engineer and former professor at Georgia Institute of Technology, determined to measure the influence of plant growth on an energy field generated by a healer at some distance away. He used a rotary electromechanical transducer and strip chart recorder in order to measure plant growth. Drs. Ambrose and Olga Worrall were asked to pray and send energy to the plants from their home in Baltimore, some six hundred miles away. During an eleven-hour period, the plants grew at the rate of 52.5 mils per hour—over eight hundred percent the normal rate!"

The Method

But *how* do you do it? As I have said before: no visualization, affirmation, or imagining of any kind is needed. Please remember this. This is the method:

(1) Be in a quiet place where you can be relaxed. Sit down if you wish.

(2) If you know where the recipient is, be facing that direction. This is helpful, but not essential.

(3) Fix firmly in your mind that you are going to treat that specific individual, that the Drawing Out or Putting In which you will be doing will "reach" that person. There is no need to visualize the person, just to hold the thought-concept that the Magnetism is effecting (as I say, *reaching*) his body.

(4) If there is a specific body part that needs help you can feel that it is being effected. Or, you can just feel that the recipient in general is being effected.

(5) Treat for as long as you like—*no time limit need be observed here.* But *do* wait seventy-two hours before treating again, except when it is an emergency where the "natural" results of non-treatment would be worse than any reactions that might be produced.

Some Pointers

Here are a couple of points from my experience with Long Distance treatment that might be useful to you.

First, I use the Putting In technique for Long Distance, since I find that it is very effective and, rather than have to think of a particular body area I can simply work with the idea that the Magnetism is reaching the recipient. And that force will go where it is needed, just as "regular" medicine affects the ill body part even though it circulates through the entire system after being swallowed or injected. Also, by just sending the Magnetism to the person's body in general, rather than thinking of a particular part, the entire system of the recipient can be benefitted, including other areas that neither I nor the recipient may know need help—but that would not receive benefit if I concentrated on just one part of the recipient's body.

Second, I have no need to visualize the person (you really don't even need to know their name) or "direct" the energy. Rather, I just position my hands; firmly set in my mind that the Magnetic current is going to the recipient; and let it flow. Every time, for me personally, I can actually feel the person's presence, right away. I prefer to work with my eyes closed so nothing visual can distract me. As a result, I feel just as if the recipient is right in the room, in front of me, and I am feeling his "vibrations" (which is in actuality his personal Magnetism). Because of this impression of "being present," no affirmation, visualization, or imagining is needed. This, I am sure, can be your experience with practice. I know this is real, because there is a big difference between imagining or remembering a person's presence and really "feeling" it. The memory or imagination of a burn, for example, is not the same thing as really getting burned! And the difference is just about as dramatic in working with the Long Distance method.

4

WhAT AbOUT CANCER?

It is said that we all get cancer—even several times—sometime in our life. But the body resists and destroys it before it is of any significant growth. Even in recognized cancer patients, what the medical profession terms "spontaneous remission" sometimes occurs. By that they mean that in some mysterious way the cancer has been dissolved. The "mysterious way" is not mysterious at all—it is simply the natural, self-healing power within the body; the power we call Magnetism.

I don't feel that I can say it any better than Dr. A.S. Raleigh, so I will quote his views on the matter:

"The proper thing to do is to bring a current of Magnetism through the body and out through this cancer [by using the Drawing Out method] . . .. Let this current of Magnetic force flowing from the body, stream out through the cancer, carrying away this waste product. . . . This cancerous tissue which is eating away and poisoning the sound tissue, must also be permeated with magnetism. . . .

"You must kill this cancerous state and remove this tissue in this Magnetic way . . .. Concentrate a strong current of vitality so as to intensely vitalize the part of the body, at the same time giving the food which will help to throw off this cancerous poison. . . .

"Be very careful in doing this. If you make the slightest slip you are liable to take the cancer yourself, because you are really drawing those forces out into your negative hand; therefore, after you have given a treatment, be sure to concentrate your force very positively and make it flow out. [See page 28] . . .

"Also, while treating a patient for cancer do not let any one else stay in the room; there is danger of giving it to others; also it is best not to treat another patient for another fifteen or twenty minutes after treating a cancerous patient, because there is danger of the evil Magnetism affecting the next patient, and the room should be fumigated with incense of a very powerful character, immediately after a treatment of that kind, so as to destroy the poison which is driven out of the system. . . .

"One thing we must call your attention to: Do not follow the practice of placing the positive hand over the cancer and directing the force inward [through the Putting In method]; that method is simply following the methods of operation which are employed by all the physicians. What you want to do is not to drive the force into the cancer, but draw the poison out of the system through the cancer, as the cancer is the effort of Nature to eliminate this waste, and we should cooperate with this effort, work in conjunction with it, and by doing this we will be able to hasten the cure."

Although I agree basically with Dr. Raleigh's statements, I do think that it could be of benefit in some applications to practice Putting In, since you would actually be enhancing the body's "fighting power" that dissolves the cancer in cases of so-called "spontaneous remission." So if you do not feel that you should take the definite risk involved in working on cancer by utilizing Drawing Out, then don't hesitate to use Putting In (*if* this does not cause the recipient's discomfort to increase).

As has been said before, Magnetic Therapy increases and stimulates that natural self-curing force within the body. So nothing could be more appropriate to utilize in cases of cancer. However I personally would never rely on Magnetic Therapy alone if I had cancer. Rather, I would utilize every aid I could find, especially those outlined in *Laetrile: Nutritional Control for Cancer with Vitamin B-17* (especially pages 283-300, "Physician's Handbook of Vitamin B-17 Therapy"),[1] *The Grape Cure*,[2] and *The Master Cleanser*.[3]

Fred Wortman's Way

Even more intriguing than the ideas in the above books is that suggested by Fred Wortman. Here it is in the words of Joseph F. Goodavage, who supplied us with the information:

"When Fred Wortman of Albany, Georgia, developed an inoperable malignance of the intestine, he faced the prospect of long treatment with x-radiation 'therapy.' 'The doctors,' Mr. Wortman said, 'refused to operate when they discovered the condition of my bank balance.'

"Being a wide reader, he remembered a simple remedy for cancer that was given in a book by a 'Mrs. Brandt,'[4] and looked it up.

"It was rather involved and cumbersome to follow, so he reduced it to its essentials, took the 'cure' and was completely cancer-free within a month.

"Wortman then had his experience published in 'The Independent' and received hundreds of replies. Over two hundred cancer sufferers reported complete cures—total recovery. The grape treatment cured lung cancer in two weeks, he reported. Cancer of the prostate took a little longer—about a month. Only four cases of leukemia (cancer of the blood) were treated, but the judicious usage of grape juice cured them all.

"Start the treatment like this:

"Begin with a twenty-four ounce bottle of (dark Concord) grape juice the first thing in the morning. Do not eat until Noon. Take a couple of swallows every ten or fifteen minutes (don't gulp it down all at once). After twelve o'clock, live the rest of the day normally, but do not eat anything after eight o'clock in the evening. . . . Food seems to carry off the curative agent in the grape juice, which may be magnesium, so stick to the fast between 8 p.m. and Noon the following day.

"Keep this up every day for two weeks to one month. . . .

"The dark Concord grape juice treatment is reported to be nearly 100% effective."

Later on Wortman collected information on four hundred cases treated successfully in this way.

Certainly, if I had cancer, I would try the above method—especially since from Noon on I could eat normally, and would not be starving myself. I suppose Mr. Wortman used bottled Concord grape juice from the local grocery store. Whether unadulterated grape juice is still available in regular grocery stores I don't know, but certainly health food stores should carry it, I would think.

Anyway, I say all this to say simply that I would not ignore other avenues of help if I should ever get cancer.

5

WHAT ABOUT

MENTAL ILLNESS?

If "only in a healthy body can you have a healthy mind," there is no reason why Magnetic Therapy could not be of help to mentally troubled or ill people just from the standpoint that it can assist the body in maintaining health. On my part, I am really convinced that a lot of mental aberration is really *physical* aberration, and modern psychiatry seems to agree—otherwise why should psychiatrists be medical doctors and not simply psychologists? Even more, I believe that confused polarity results in mental confusion and may even, if serious enough, produce "insane" behavior. Previously I have told my experience in having my own polarity confused. I believe that if a person underwent what I did—though to a much greater degree and for a prolonged time—he could not help but "get peculiar" from just the weirdness of feeling and mental confusion that he might experience. Often we hear of cases where a person has undergone a "traumatic" experience, and then developed mental problems. Emotional shock especially causes confusion—and even reversal—of polarity. Any person who has experienced a shock of any kind—physical or mental—should have their polarity checked and corrected. Accidents also produce confused polarity, as a rule. Anything that jolts the system either mentally or physically (since they cannot be separated) can upset the Magnetic flow in our bodies.

Not to suggest that teen-agers are crazy, but you may find that Magnetic Therapy can be of great help in those years when so much nervous instability and emotional growing pains manifest themselves.

The elderly also, who so often are labeled as senile or suffering from "old age," may be found to simply have confused polarity.

I am certainly not suggesting that you start working with the mentally disturbed to the exclusion of qualified professional help for them; but I do think that Magnetic therapy could certainly speed their recovery, and you should not hesitate to use it for their benefit.

6

INCREASING

YOUR MAGNETISM

The more magnetic you are, the more efficiently and effectively you can apply Magnetic Therapy. Some people, in fact, must increase their magnetism just to minimally apply it—their natural magnetism is so weak. But everyone who wants to seriously work with Magnetism should strive to be as magnetic as possible. The following are some ways in which I believe you can markedly enhance your magnetism.

Diet

I hesitate to write anything on this, as everybody seems to think his way of eating is the only way—and that is mistaken. Different people need differing diets. Just because a certain dietary regimen has helped one person is no sign it will be good for *us*. And simply because an exponent of a particular "diet" is healthy may only mean that he is so healthy he can survive it—and we might not! So please understand that in this matter I am only giving personal opinions and I am keenly aware that my ideas might not be good for some people. "Diet craze" is a curse, and I have never seen true health result from it, because any obsession is bad for the mind and body.

The body tissues and nerves are the receptacles and instruments of Magnetism, and their condition can be either more or less conducive to Magnetism depending on their condition. The body is not just a magnet, it is an *electrical* magnet—we can even say it is a *battery*. And just as certain chemical solutions are needed to run a battery, so a certain body chemistry is needed for magnetic efficiency.

A diet completely free from meat, fish, eggs, or anything that contains them to any degree is the most desirable, I feel. For twenty years I have not eaten meat, fish, or eggs, and the benefits have been so evident that meat-eating seems to me the utmost folly—so much so, that I hesitate to write about it lest I be too overbearing on the subject. This I can say: every doctor the members of our Monastery have consulted has told us

55

that we are the healthiest people they ever encounter. One widely known diagnostician referred to those he has examined as "shockingly healthy." A heart specialist has even asked for the recipes we use in our Monastery so he can pass them on to his patients, for he says that our cholesterol levels, condition of blood and internal organs, is perfect. For centuries monks have had the reputation of living long and not showing their age. And monks have always abstained from meat, fish, and eggs. Your local health food store should be able to supply you with books by others much more qualified than I am to discuss the matter "scientifically," so I won't burden these pages or you with facts and figures on this subject. I do recommend that you read *The Master Cleanser*,[3] *The Health Secrets of a Naturopathic Doctor*,[5] and *The Vegetarian's Self-defense Manual*[6] about this. And there are other good books available through health stores, especially those distributed by Nutri-Books Corporation.

Just A Little More!

Let me pound the soap box just a little on this, however. First of all, Magnetism is not electricity. Therefore, although electricity is all the same quality, no matter how it is generated, Magnetism varies. It carries with it the qualities of its source. The body is an energy extractor (much more impressive and efficient than an atomic reactor), and just as a loom can weave many types of thread into cloth that differs according to the type and origin of the thread, so the energy-magnetism of the body and mind is conditioned by food. "Psychology Today" had a brief article in one issue about a man who is seriously studying the fact that people take on the traits of the type of animals whose flesh they predominantly eat! Especially he was interested in the "chickenness" of people who eat a lot of chicken. (By the way, even *sterile* eggs have been found to register the heartbeat rate of the chicken embryo—so that Magnetism is there, also.) Joseph F. Goodavage's book: *Magic, Science of the Future*,[7] contains amazing information about the "L-fields" which surround bodies. This subtle energy affects the mind of a person who eats meat. Just as the physical energy of the animal is absorbed into the body, the magnetic and mental energies are also absorbed into the magnetism and mind of the person who eats that animal's flesh. That is my experience and observation.

But Why Vegetables?

Since plants are hardly as developed as animals, why, then, should their consumption be preferable? This has been shown in just the last decade or so with experiments that have definitely established that plants

56

can pick up thoughts—are telepathic. The psychic sensitivity of plants exceeds that of animals. The simple thought about destroying a plant produces an intense reaction in that plant, but a similar thought directed toward a cow, chicken, pig, or fish would produce no such reaction. Why? Because their Magnetism is much less sensitive. So a *sensible* vegetarian diet can certainly increase the sensitivity of the mind and the facility of thought. The Magnetism of plants is "lighter," more malleable, so the mind can absorb it easily and shape it, so to speak. The Magnetism of animals is heavy, dull, and tends to effect the mind of the eater, rather than the other way around (no matter what Cayce supposedly said). It is my observation that a vegetarian is much quicker in mind than a meat-eater, and positively much more capable of subtle, abstract thought. Plant Magnetism is also more near the "pure" form of Magnetism which vivifies the universe, so the physical organism nourished on that type of Magnetism will more easily respond to and convey that Magnetism which we are dealing with in Magnetic Therapy.

Good Sense Is Needed

One last word on this: a sensible diet is the secret. Nutrition should be studied. Every person—vegetarian or not—should have access to *Nutrition Almanac.* [8] This gives the needed information to formulate a practical diet for yourself. Two other good books are: *Diet For a Small Planet,* [9] and *Recipes For a Small Planet.* [10] Don't believe the food-fad books, or believe that there is "the right diet" for the whole world that will work miracles. No. Find your own. And in the main I think you will find that a good vegetarian diet will improve both your health and your Magnetism.

What You Wear

Strange as it may seem, the wearing of *copper rings* on the ring fingers can increase your Magnetism to a marked degree. The rings should not be just any kind, but a particular type. They should be formed from heavy copper wire (No. 10 gauge is the best). The ring for your positive hand should be formed of a copper wire fashioned into two circular loops, wound clockwise, if viewed as being wound *away* from you. The ring for your negative hand should be formed of a copper wire fashioned into three circular loops, wound counterclockwise, if viewed as being wound away from you (see Fig. 30). Why copper, and why the differing number of loops for the hands? I

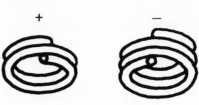

Fig. 30

don't know. Any explanation I might give would only be an ignorant guess. I am sure a plausible explanation could be formulated and sound very "scientific," but what value would it have? What really counts is that every person I have worked with has had the Magnetism of their hands increased by nearly one hundred percent by the wearing of these rings. That's enough for me.

Someone who has a ring mandrel can make them for you if he knows your ring size. The copper wire can be gotten from a hardware or electrical supply store in the form of "solid copper electrical wire" (you will need to remove the insulation). Some crafts and jeweler's supply stores sell the right kind of copper wire, as well. If you want a ring mandrel of your own you can no doubt get one from a jeweler's supply company.

You can either only wear the rings while working on people, or wear them all the time.

Body Cleanliness

Not just soap-and-water cleanliness, but internal cleanliness. For this read *The Master Cleanser*, already mentioned. I could give a condensation of the routine in this book, but I am afraid that I might omit something important. This book is a must for anyone interested in good health. What it recommends will be a great help in increasing Magnetism.

Breathing

Before now I have likened the flow of Magnetism in the body to breathing. In reality, there is a fundamental connection between our breathing and the flow of Magnetism through our body. The Magnetism can be increased and even controlled through breathing. This is how the Indian yogis attain such complete control over their vital functions—even learning to live without the means of external breathing. This I don't recommend to you! But there is a breathing exercise which is most beneficial in regulating, balancing, and increasing Magnetic flow. It is called *Nadi Shuddhi*, which literally means "Nerve Cleaning" and is meant to clear and tone up the subtle channels of the body through which Magnetism flows. Here it is:

(1) Sit comfortably and be relaxed.

(2) With your right thumb, close your right nostril by pressing on its side (not by sticking your thumb in the nostril).

(3) Inhale calmly and steadily through your left nostril, until your lungs are comfortably full (no need to strain them).

(4) Then, with the ring finger and little finger of your right hand, close the left nostril by pressing on the side of the nose; and move your thumb

away from your right nostril so it can open.

(5) Exhale steadily and fully (no need for strain here, either) through your right nostril.

(6) Inhale steadily and fully through the right nostril; then close that nostril with your thumb as before.

(7) Exhale through your left nostril, removing your fingers.

These six steps constitute one cycle. Do four cycles of this, three times a day. It may not seem like very many times, but if you practice regularly you will come to see the profound effect it can have. If after a few months of practice you want to increase the amount of cycles, do so, but carefully and slowly. Please note that you do not hold the breath at any time.

A Second Exercise

Here is another method that differs quite a bit from the one above, but has a value of its own. Transcendental Meditation or the Relaxation Response cannot touch it for either effectiveness or benefits to be gained. It can be your nervous system's best friend, when done correctly.

(1) Sit quietly and be relaxed. Have your mouth closed, so you will breathe only through the nose.

(2) Be aware of your breath. Just "watch" as it flows in and out naturally. No special control of breathing is needed.

(3) As your breath flows in naturally, mentally say the syllable: **HUNG** (as in "I *hung* the picture"). Say it only once, "lazily," so it stretches out through the duration of the inhalation. In other words, if your breath is long and slow, then you will say: H-H-H-U-U-U-N-N-N-G-G-G; letting it sound like a smooth gong, the duration of your breath. If, however, your inhaling may be short, you will say it briefly.

(4) As your breath flows out naturally, mentally say the syllable: **SUH** (as in a theatrical Southern accent: "Colonel, *Suh*"). It, too, should be expanded to fit the duration of your exhalation: S-S-S-U-U-U-H-H-H.

(5) Continue saying HUNG and SUH in keeping with your breath, letting the syllables match the breath (not the other way round).

(6) Do this for ten or fifteen minutes in the beginning, at least twice a day. Then increase it to thirty minutes a session if you have the time. The more you practice the more effective each subsequent session will be. Simple as it is, it is also profound in effect. You should only do it when sitting and relaxed. When active, do not do it.

Energizing Exercise

To greatly—and consciously—increase your Magnetism, the following exercise is most effective.

(a) Upon awakening in the morning, remain in bed, lying on your back with your eyes closed. Then think of your body as divided into twenty parts:

(1) Left foot	(11) Left forearm
(2) Right foot	(12) Right forearm
(3) Left calf	(13) Left upper arm
(4) Right calf	(14) Right upper arm
(5) Left thigh	(15) Left chest
(6) Right thigh	(16) Right chest
(7) Left hip	(17) Left of neck
(8) Right hip	(18) Right of neck
(9) Abdomen	(19) Front of neck
(10) Stomach	(20) Back of neck

(b) Tense all these twenty parts simultaneously, hold the tension for a count of three, and then quickly relax and exhale through your mouth. Relax completely, not moving a muscle, but feel as though all tension is leaving your body and you are "melting" into peacefulness. For as long as is comfortable, remain without breathing.

(c) Now gently and individually tense and relax each of the above twenty body parts.

(d) Then practice "cumulative relaxation" as follows:

Placing your attention on the instep of your left foot, slowly tense the entire foot—gently and smoothly moving from low to high tension. Draw your toes under while doing this. (If your foot tends to develop muscle cramps, you can curl the toes upward rather than under.)

Keeping the tension at high in your left foot, tense your right foot in the same manner. Holding the tension in that foot also, continue to proceed upwards, tensing each of the twenty body parts—while retaining the tension in the parts previously tensed. Keep each part tensed as you move on carefully to the succeeding parts, as follows:

(1) Left foot	(9) Abdomen (area below
(2) Right foot	the navel)
(3) Left calf	(10) Stomach (area above
(4) Right calf	the navel)
(5) Left thigh	(11) Left forearm
(6) Right thigh	(12) Right forearm
(7) Left hip	(13) Left upper arm
(8) Right hip	(14) Right upper arm

(15) Left chest	(18) Right of neck
(16) Right chest	(19) Front of neck
(17) Left of neck	(20) Back of neck

Gently increase the tension simultaneously in all the body parts, and vibrate the entire body, holding the breath for a count of six—high tension being maintained in all twenty parts. BE SURE ALL PARTS ARE TENSED.

Exhale completely—and through the mouth—and carefully relax the body parts, in reverse order—from neck to feet. (When doing this exercise sitting or standing, upon exhalation drop your chin to your chest, simultaneously relaxing the front, back, left and right sides of your neck.) Continue relaxing one part at a time. Be sure the tension in each body part is maintained until its turn to be relaxed. If while relaxing a part you find that you have involuntarily relaxed a lower part whose turn for relaxation should be later, tense that part and keep relaxing in the correct order.

(e) Getting up from bed, do the entire process of part "(d)" *twice*.

This may be done any time you feel tired or nervous—but should especially be done every day upon awakening.

Regulation of Life

Magnetism and life energy are inseparable. So obviously the more you expend your energy, the less Magnetic you will be. What Jesus terms "riotous living" (Luke 15:13), weakens and debilitates the nervous system, rendering a person incapable of effectively applying Magnetism, and certainly makes it difficult for him to even benefit by it as a recipient. A sober, moral life is essential for those who would benefit themselves and others through Magnetism. This is especially true in the department of sex.

Dr. A.S. Raleigh wrote: "It is, consequently by the polarizing of those forces which are ordinarily sent forth to one of the opposite sex, by polarizing them and bringing them back up into our own being, restoring them to the brain, that the regeneration of the body is made possible. The sexual principle is, therefore, the great healing force of the human organism and should be employed intelligently as a healing agent; but to do this it is necessary to lead a pure life. It is for this reason that celibates are able to do much more effective healing than married men and women or than people who do not lead perfectly chaste lives. If they do not lead lives of perfect purity, they will transmit what force they have, of course, but it will not be anything like as effective—may, in fact, rob them of energy they require."

While we hear a lot of admiring words about the "healing temples" of ancient Egypt and Greece, one cardinal fact is ignored: the healers in those shrines were vowed to celibacy. Even pagan Rome recognized that virginity had a unique spiritual power—the prayers and worship of the Vestal Virgins were considered of more effect than those of all the rest of the Empire.

However, I am not telling you to be a monk or nun. A sensibly controlled sex life (something even "the doctors" used to advocate not so long ago—remember when?) *is* important for you. Isn't it significant that the rate of disease and insanity has increased in proportion as permissiveness and the "new morality" has arisen more and more? I believe it is directly related. And so does Dr. Edwin Flatto, whose book, *Warning: Sex May Be Hazardous To Your Health,*[11] is an invaluable source of information (including Sigmund Freud's real ideas on celibacy) for those with enough character and nerve to "take it."

Actually, all-around healthful living is necessary for successful work with Magnetism. Live healthily, and you will be able to help others to health—it *should* be contagious!

Prayer

I have no hesitation in saying that *prayer* is a great enhancement of your life, and of course of Magnetism. During our first session with Ina she stated: "If you aren't a praying person when you start this work, *you will be* later on." I believe it.

As we have seen, for correct practice of Magnetic Therapy no "mind work" is needed. And detachment is best. So instead of standing or sitting with empty minds, if we fill our minds with aspiration to the One Healer we will find the real secret of health for our minds and souls as well as for our bodies and those of others. The recipient, too, who prays will find this to be so. While Magnetic Therapy is not "spiritual" or "divine" healing, it still is—like everything in existence—a part of the *life* which has God as its sole Source and Support. And the closer anything is to that Source, the better and more meaningful it is.

There is no need for many words and sentences in prayer. The simple name of **Jesus** is best of all, I find. And even silent aspiration and "reaching out" of the mind toward God is of effect. Those who try will not be disappointed.

Leslie O. Korth gives this example in his book, *Healing Magnetism*: "When, about twenty years ago, Dr. Fritsche had the first opportunity to experience healing magnetism, having devoted much time and study to it, he became acquainted with two doctors, each seventy years of age, who themselves were masters of the art. One was abounding in energy and geniality, whose magnetic powers were very much in evidence. The other was a practitioner of a religious nature for whom, in theory as well as practice, life's power and God's power were one and the same thing. Both doctors enjoyed outstanding successes in the magnetic treatment of the sick. The difference between them, in their respective practices, lay in the first one becoming exhausted by his treatment, whilst the other practitioner found that the more magnetism he gave out, the more it increased in himself, as the magnetism was not coming from him but through him from the cosmos, with the result that his efforts did not leave him in a state of fatigue."

Another expert has written: "The nearer you are in consciousness to the Source of all Power, the greater will be your healing power. Remember always that back of all the Power of the Universe is that Infinite Power, which is the source of all Power and Energy. Remember that you are as a particle of this one Infinite life, and that all that is Real about you is so because of your relationship with that Infinite Being. Try to realize this fully, and you will find that with the recognition will come a strength and power far surpassing anything that you have before known, or acquired by any other means. This is the source of all real power, and it is open to him or her who seeks it."

"The injury done by separating the religious spirit from the magnetic act is incalculable"—so says the anonymous author of *Vital Magnetic Cure.*[12]

Although this chapter was written with the operator in mind, it applies to the recipient as well.

7

ThINGS ThAT DECREASE OR UNBALANCE YOUR MAGNETISM

Already we have discussed some things—such as metal and leather—that decrease or interrupt the movement of Magnetism. But let's consider a few more.

Leather and You

Leather seems to act as an inhibitor of Magnetic flow—perhaps it has an insulating property, or perhaps it retains some Magnetic field of its own, since it is the skin of a once-living animal (just like the sterile eggs). Anyhow, a leather belt will certainly cut down the Magnetic flow of the operator in applying Magnetic Therapy. So when you work on someone, try to have a non-leather belt for the time of treatment. The recipient, too, should remove his belt if it is leather. (Whether, then, a person should wear a leather belt at all is a good question; since if it does inhibit Magnetic flow it cannot be good to wear one all day long. This may be why the yogis of India prohibited leather, and not from principles of non-violence.) The same applies to leather shoes. If convenient, wear some type of cloth or canvas shoes (house slippers are fine) when doing the Magnetic work. And certainly the recipient should remove his shoes if they are leather. The shoe matter, though, is not as important as the belt. I have worked with leather shoes on, and though it does lessen the effectiveness of the treatment slightly, it in no way has the effect of a leather belt on the operator's ability.

Synthetic Fabrics

As we have discussed before, the wearing of wool and silk (and perhaps some synthetic fabrics) hinders the flow of Magnetism. It has even been suggested by some researchers on Magnetism that wearing some types of synthetic materials is injurious to the health. If so, might it be because of the fabrics' effect on the body Magnetism?

Jewelry

Since, as also discussed previously, metal jewelry inhibits Magnetic flow in therapy, there is good reason to suppose that such metal jewelry causes irregularity in the Magnetic circulation in the body at all times, and therefore may cause blockages, leaks, or "low voltage" in the body parts contacted—even through a layer or two of clothing. Am I suggesting that you throw your jewelry away? Not at all; but I do suggest that once you have developed your Magnetic sensitivity, you test whether or not some pieces of your jewelry might not effect the circulation of Magnetism in your body. I personally refuse to wear a wristwatch for this reason. When I was about junior-high school age, I was given a beautiful gold wristwatch with an expandable metal band. By the time I reached high school I observed that the part of my arm where I wore the watch was smaller than the corresponding part on the opposite arm. I quit wearing the watch, and in a couple of years or so that part of my arm was of equal size with the other. At that time I attributed it to the pressure of the watch band on my arm. But after learning about Magnetism I have concluded that the metal band inhibited the normal flow of Magnetism to that body part, and thus inhibited its growth and development. I may be wrong, but why take a chance?

Hypnotism

Never let yourself be hypnotized. If a doctor recommends it, get another doctor. If a psychiatrist recommends it, ask if there are any possible alternatives. Hypnotism is very little understood, so I am not able to give any "why"—but it creates a static condition in the Magnetism that should be flowing evenly through your body. Any kind of induced "trance" has a negative effect on you in the long run. Don't.

Zone Therapy/Reflexology

The type of Zone Therapy (Reflexology) in which the operator puts pressure on areas of the foot and pokes or gouges those areas, is extremely detrimental to the body's Magnetism, and throws off its normal circulation. The temporary (and therefore false) relief given by such a system of Zone Therapy is bought at too dear a price.

Treatment With Magnets

Like so many other things, magnets can be used to benefit—but not in the long run. It is easy to see that a magnet applied to the body would tend to polarize the body's Magnetism to flow toward it. But for health, Magnetism must circulate from the positive to the negative poles of the body without interruption. The side effects of treatment with magnets is not worth it. Furthermore, the magnetism put out by a piece of metal or plastic is just not the same as the Magnetism of your body. It is similar, but it is not the same. And your body needs a force in total compatibility with it for efficient healing. Magnetic Therapy as given in this book supplies exactly that.

Modern Acupuncture

"Modern" acupuncture means acupuncture which uses electrical currents. The traditional acupuncture is wonderful, and there is no complaint about that. But researchers have found that the electrified kind can really wreak havoc with your Magnetism. I have had just one acupuncture treatment which involved electricity, and that was enough! The effect was drastic, and not worth the little benefit received. One person being treated in the enclosure just next to me began to faint dead away after a few seconds of the treatment. No thanks.

Electric Shocks

If you get an electrical shock, then have your polarity corrected immediately.

X-Rays

Sometimes we all have to get X-rayed. So when you do, right away have your polarity checked and corrected if need be, and Draw Out from the area (if that area was worked on in *less* than seventy-two hours, then Draw Out for just three to five minutes).

Television

If you sit too close to a television set—especially a color set—you are bombarded with harmful radiations, one side effect being imbalancing and making "static" your Magnetism. Be careful, and find out how far away the manufacturer recommends you should sit for viewing to be safe.

Fluorescent Lights

Studies have shown that prolonged exposure to fluorescent lights can be detrimental to your health. Avoid all use of such lights whenever possible.

Kirilian Photography

There has understandably been a great interest in this method of studying the subtle Magnetic radiations of the body. But it has been found that elements in the bone structure of the body can be damaged by such high frequency bombardment as is required for the production of the photographs.

Insecticides and Detergents

Insecticides adversely affect your body's Magnetism. Even more common a culprit is the detergent you use daily. The prolonged use of detergents in dishwashing, hand laundering, etc., can completely inhibit the Magnetic flow within the hands. Since you "breathe in" your negative hand, and "breathe out" your positive hand, you can imagine the effect on your body of those channels being blocked! And that raises another question: what about the continual use of body soaps that contain detergent? Most *do* contain detergents, and some even advertise themselves as "detergent bars." Caution is needed here, too.

Comfrey

Mrs. Francis Nixon and her fellow-researchers have discovered that tea made from Comfrey *leaves* causes a static condition in the Magnetism of the bones in the mouth, throat, and upper chest. Whether the Comfrey root also has this effect is not yet known. Even "natural" medicines can have unhappy side-effects. That is why I stick to "Nature's own": Magnetism.

Drugs

"Here the mischief of giving morphine was evident—*it prevented the full effects of magnetism for days"* (Mesmer).

Both illegal drugs—such as LSD and Marijuana—and legal ones (medicines) can play havoc with your body's Magnetism. Most should never be used, and the others should be avoided whenever possible (watch those additives and preservatives in your daily food, too).

Tobacco and alcoholic beverages are drugs, also. Nicotine is a harmful drug (poisonous, actually), and alcohol is a poison to the system—physical, mental and moral. Those who smoke or "drink" are filled with toxins and deranged Magnetism. Even the "light" users of those things, as well as the "heavies." NEVER should they attempt to apply Magnetic Therapy, for they will transfer the negative Magnetism in their bodies to the recipient's body. And they will be much harder to work on as recipients. I would almost never Draw Out from smokers or drinkers, or apply the Short

Circuit on them. The Body Sweep and Putting In are the only processes I would use.

8

OVERCOMING
A STATIC CONDITION

You may find that for some unknown reason your own Magnetism will just quit flowing to any marked degree (of course, it doesn't really stop altogether), and you cannot apply Magnetic Therapy to others.

Sometimes this is our own Magnetic system warning us that we are not in good enough physical condition to apply Magnetism just at that time. It is a safety device. So if, after trying the things I am going to suggest in this chapter, your Magnetism is still in a (nearly) "static" condition, then accept it and "take off" a few days until you find your Magnetism flowing again normally.

As soon as you get into the static condition, have your polarity checked. This may be the problem. But if your polarity is just fine (but weak), try these three following methods (one may be sufficient):

Vitalization Stance

Remove your shoes. Stand upright and raise your arms out and level with your shoulders so you are standing in the form of a Cross. Face either East or West, so the fingers of your positive hand are pointing South and the fingers of your negative hand are pointing North.

The palm of your positive hand should be turned down, and the palm of your negative hand should be turned up. Then cup your hands and fingers so the fingertips are pointing up (negative hand) and down (positive hand)—see Fig. 31.

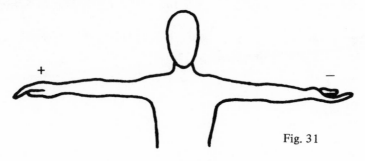

Fig. 31

Stand in this way, relaxed for a few minutes, and be attentive to the feelings of Magnetic flow in your hands. If your arms get tired, stop for a while and then resume the Stance. Three to five minutes should be enough, but if after ten or fifteen minutes there is no increase in your Magnetic flow, then do the next method.

It is important to remain as relaxed as possible when doing this.

Salt and Soda Bath

One of the best Magnetic therapists of the last century was Colonel Olcott, co-founder of the Theosophical Society. The cures he worked in Ceylon and India were astonishing to all (including himself, at first!). He writes in his memoirs, *Old Diary Leaves*, that at times he, too, experienced a static condition in his Magnetism. At such times, when he was in Ceylon, he would go for a swim in the ocean. Emerging from the ocean, he would find himself revitalized and ready to go back to more treatment.

Mrs. Francis Nixon, in her admirable work on energies, discovered that a bath in a solution of sea salt and soda was able to correct static conditions in the Magnetism. Here is how to do it.

Dissolve one pound of sea salt (most health food stores carry it—but be sure there are no additives) and one pound of baking soda in a bathtub of lukewarm water not hotter than 90-98 degrees. Submerge your whole body in this solution, and soak for about ten minutes, immersing your head, as well, for short intervals. Be sure your shoulders are completely submerged. Have a similar solution in a water glass, and rinse your mouth out with it a few times, as well. *Only you who are taking the bath should stir the salt and soda into the water with your own hands.*

Feet In Earth

Something that is very helpful to the increase and balance of Magnetism (even if your Magnetic flow is all right) is to go outside in the early morning just before dawn, dig out a small cavity and stand in it, *facing toward the rising sun*, covering your feet back up with the earth. Stand there as the sun rises (you might try the Vitalization Stance while doing this).

Another good practice is to walk barefoot on the dew and grass at sunrise. This is a good thing to do anytime.

9

MAGNETIC AIDS TO HEALTH

This chapter, like the last ones, applies to recipients as well as operators. The two hands are the best "instruments" for health. But certain mechanical aids are helpful—especially for those who do not have someone to treat them. The following are aids I have personally found to be of value—all related to Magnetic Therapy.

Spoon Rub

A Body Sweep is one of the best things to get the Magnetism flowing unhindered through the body. But if you have no one to do a Body Sweep, a Spoon Rub can be next best.

Take a *stainless steel* spoon and rub the bottoms of your feet, including the toes. In the feet are nerve endings—plexii—connected to the glands and organs of the body. The contact of the stainless steel pulls the current through the nerve endings and this in turn stimulates the entire nervous system and helps tone up the body processes.

A Spoon Rub over the entire body—negative side to positive side, beginning at the feet—is also helpful.

Even better than a spoon is a steel roller bearing—since it contains more steel and thus has greater drawing power.

Vitic

This is truly amazing. Egyptian statues show both pharoahs and priests holding a rod in each hand. This intrigued A.B. Baines, who did research on what the rods might have been—and for what purpose. He came to the conclusion that one rod was of carbon and the other of magnetic ore (lodestone). The purpose was to increase vitality and Magnetism, he decided. Therefore he began to experiment with this force, which he called "Vitic." From his research and that of others a device was evolved which can be of tremendous help in increasing vitality and the general condition of the body—especially the internal organs.

A Vitic Device consists of two horseshoe magnets (Alnico magnets are preferred) strong enough to lift thirty-two pounds or more, a copper-coated steel rod seven-eighths of an inch in diameter, and a carbon rod

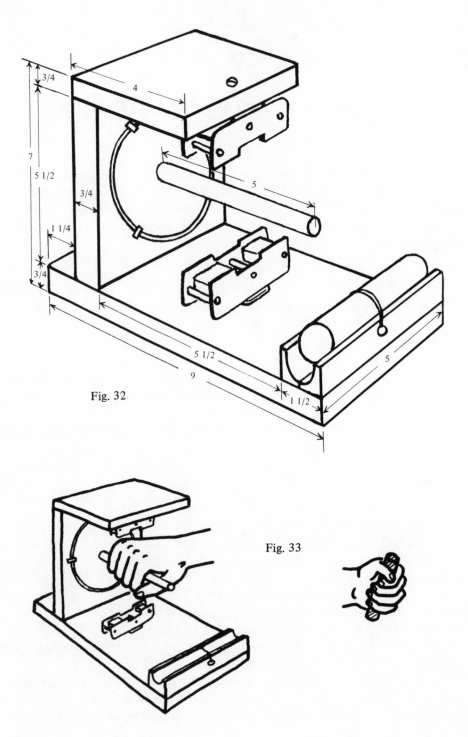

Fig. 32

Fig. 33

one inch to one-and-a-half inches in diameter. The two magnets should be mounted so they are pointing at each other, the opposite poles facing. Between them—so as to be in the center of the magnetic field from the two magnets—should be the steel rod. An illustration with measurements is given (see Fig. 32). An overlapping loop of twelve-gauge, or heavier, copper wire completes the device (this enhances the effect, but is not essential).

The carbon rod is held in one hand, and the steel rod in the other (see Fig. 33). That is all.

What happens? According to Baines, "Hard Carbon such as is used in arc lamps will give out a certain amount of force which, experience has taught us, is not to be distinguished from nerve force." So the carbon acts as an antenna to bring magnetic force into the body. The steel rod stimulates this action and heightens the Magnetic level.

Dr. J. Horne Wilson, writing in "The Practitioner" of June, 1914, stated: "I may mention that a rod of carbon, . . . has a most remarkable effect on body deflection . . .. If held in contact with the right side of the body for five or ten minutes it makes the hand-to-hand deflection strongly positive, and has exactly the opposite effect if held on the left side of the body.

"This force has a marked influence on the electrical condition of the body . . .. It evidently charges the body with a force akin to nerve energy, as it is retained for a much longer period than electricity is."

Dr. White-Robertson, in *Studies in Electro-Pathology*, says: "We have been able to observe gratifying changes in cases of breakdown apparently by increasing the nerve charge through the new carbons. What this force is, we do not as yet know, nor is it known to the eminent physiologist to whom we have demonstrated it . . .. [It] is, as registered by the galvanometer over a period of twelve hours, stored probably in the unipolar ganglia of the nervous system."

More from Dr. Wilson ("Medical Times," July 25, 1914): "This form of energy will restore nerve currents to normal. The [carbon] rod held in the right hand acts as a stimulant without any depressing effect and in the left hand as a sedative. Under the stimulating influence, the nervous system is generally benefited, mental fatigue rapidly disappears and morbid conditions such as neurasthenia, insomnia and feeble action of heart yield readily."

Electronic measurement has shown that the organs and systems of the body steadily increase in vitality with regular use of the Vitic. It has been estimated that only four to eight days of regular Vitic use are needed to bring the organs and systems up to normal level.

Using the illustration, you should be able to make—or have made—your own Vitic device.

A plating company should be able to copper-plate the steel rod for you. An alternative is to paint the rod with copper or bronze paint that has genuine metal particles in it.

Magnets—Alnico or permanent ceramic magnets—can be obtained from:

Edmund Scientific
101 E. Gloucester Pike
Barrington, New Jersey 08007

Copper wire for the loop can be gotten from any hardware or electrical supply company.

If you are unable to make your own Vitic Device, you may order one from: Borderland Sciences Research Foundation, P.O. Box 548, Vista, CA 92083. From the same people you can get a most informative booklet entitled: *Vitic or Magnetic Vitality*, which contains more about the Vitic Device and its nature.

Here is the basic outline for using the Vitic Device:

(a) Remove the keepers from the magnets (if Alnico—ceramic magnets do not need keepers) when using, and replace them when finished.

(b) Hold the carbon rod in one hand, the steel rod in the other—what effect you desire determines which hands should hold what rods.

(c) Hold the rods for fifteen minutes, as a rule, but you can increase or decrease the time, as you like.

Do this twice a day, at intervals of twelve hours, if possible.

(d) For vitality, the steel rod should be held in your negative hand, and the carbon rod in your positive hand.

(e) For removing excess activity from the system the steel rod should be held in your positive hand and the carbon rod in your negative hand.

(f) Common problems where the steel rod should be held in your negative hand and the carbon rod in your positive hand: Low blood pressure; nervous breakdown; paralysis; debility; tired feeling in body and mind; marasmus; generalized weakness; to retain youthfulness.

(g) Common problems where the steel rod is held in your positive hand and the carbon rod in your negative hand: High blood pressure; palpitation of heart; diabetes mellitus; arthritis, rheumatism; insomnia; fever; excessive anger; etc.

(h) If holding the rods produces agitation or discomfort, try shifting the rods to opposite hands. Sometimes "trouble spots" will ache a little as they are being "worked on." This is all right.

(i) Always be relaxed during the treatment. Do not grip the rods tightly or squeeze them.

The main power in the Vitic seems to be in the carbon rod—the steel rod and magnets being needed to activate, balance, and direct it.

Eeman Screens

Although Eeman Screens work with Magnetism also, they are very different from the Vitic—neither can substitute for the other.

Eeman Screens are named after L.E. Eeman, who developed them. They are extremely simple. A set of Eeman Screens consists of two rectangles of copper wire screen (many believe that any type of metal will work, but we stick to copper), such as is used in windows. We use 12"x16" rectangles. Each screen has a length (about four feet) of insulated copper wire soldered to one corner. The other end of each copper wire is soldered to a four-inch length of copper tubing (one-half inch diameter works well). And that is all (seé Fig. 34). The sides of the rectangles are usually edged with cloth tape, such as is used for mending books, carpets, or upholstery, so they will not pull apart or prick the person using them.

Their use is also simple. You lie down. One screen is placed under your head, and the other beneath the base of your spine. Then the handle connected to the screen under your head is held in your left hand. In your right hand you hold the handle that is connected to the screen beneath the base of your spine. This is called "the relaxation circuit" (see Fig. 35).

Lay there, completely relaxed and at ease, your hands holding the handles, at your sides. *Cross your feet at the ankles.* This "closes the circuit." If your feet are not crossed the Screens do not work. This is an essential point. About thirty minutes, twice a day, "in circuit" is generally sufficient for a definite problem. Once a day should be enough for healthy people.

Relaxation is the key. The more relaxed you are, the better it will work.

Notice, I mentioned left and right hands for this, not positive and negative. Why? Because Eeman found that it works the same way for both left-handed and right-handed people . . . *usually.* There are exceptions. The way that works for a right-hander works fine for me, however.

In the use of Eeman Screens, unlike the Vitic, there is only one right way. If you hold the handles opposite to what I have described, you create what Eeman called "the tension circuit." You will not be able to stand it for long. Eeman never found anyone who could stand to remain in the tension circuit—even on a bet! So if holding the handles

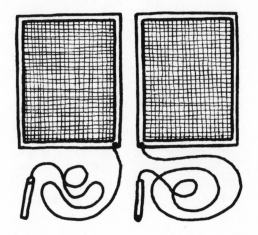

Fig. 34

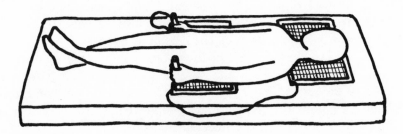

Fig. 35

Fig. 36

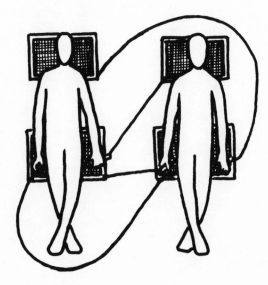

76

opposite to my description above relaxes and soothes you, then go right ahead. For you that is the correct way.

What do the Eeman Screens "do"? They correct polarity, balance and stimulate Magnetic flow. That I know. But I believe they have a great beneficial effect that goes far beyond that. And I have no explanation for it. Eeman claimed that even some emotional disorders could be alleviated by use of the Screens. I believe it. When "in circuit," people experience differing reactions. Some feel nothing for a long while, and some feel a reaction quickly. I feel marvelously relaxed and have a deep sense of tranquility and well-being. If there are any trouble spots in my body, they may ache for a while. This is because they are being worked on.

Many people fall asleep while "in circuit." This is very good.

An advantage to Eeman Screens is that they are not affected by layers of cloth, so you can put them on your mattress beneath your bedclothes and keep them there permanently—just being sure they are positioned rightly. Even a pillow can be placed between your head and the top screen.

Truly, I feel that every person should have his own set of Screens and use them regularly. When I think of their benefit to me I can't help but wonder what would result if they were used in mental hospitals, not to mention "regular" hospitals.

You should be able to make yourself a set of Screens easily. A drawing of them in detail is given. If you cannot make your own Screens, they may be obtained from Borderland Sciences Research Foundation (see page 74). Borderland also sells a booklet on the Screens entitled: *Cooperative Healing*.

Eeman recommended that the Screens be used for "team treatment" to a great extent. An illustration of that is also given (see Fig. 36). All it really amounts to is that you hold the leads of the other person's Screens in your hands—their top Screen's handle in your left, and the handle from their bottom Screen in your right (unless for you it is the opposite). Notice in the illustration that the wires *never* cross the people's bodies, but loop around them. To manage this, the two sets of Screens will need varying lengths of wire. That is: two of the four Screens will have wires four feet in length; one Screen (for the head of the person on the left) will need an eight-foot wire; and one Screen (for the base of the spine on the person on the right) will need a twelve-foot length of wire.

Team treatment with Eeman Screens definitely increases their effectiveness, and I certainly recommend it. But "solo flights" are great also.

When using either the Vitic or the Eeman Screens you should not be touching metal or—in Vitic—be sitting on a metal chair. Otherwise the effect can be neutralized. I once lay "in circuit" with Eeman Screens for nearly thirty minutes with no results because one of my feet was touching a metal bar at the foot of the bed—even though a blanket was between my foot and the bar.

Sleeping

I really don't know where to put this bit of information, so it will have to go in here.

Never sleep with your head to the North—that is, with your feet "facing" the South and your head "pointed" toward the North. This tends to reverse and confuse your polarity.

Any other direction for sleeping is fine. But sleeping with your feet toward the North and your head at the South is the most beneficial for health, according to some. This is my favorite, as well.

I have seen several people relieved of nervous problems and unexplained tension, just by shifting their sleeping position.

Magnetized Water

Magnetized water can be of great benefit, especially for the person who has no one to give them Magnetic Therapy. Magnetize a glass or cup of water simply by Putting In for several minutes. Or, you can also do a Short Circuit, holding your slightly cupped hands opposite to each other, an inch or so away from the sides of the glass or cup. Then drink it, or give it to another person. Many years ago, when Magnetism was completely unknown to me, an elderly lady in Missouri told me that she had once been cured of excruciating headaches when a friend of her father's "hypnotized" a glass of water and had her drink it. At the time she told me, it made no sense to me at all. But now, with my understanding about Magnetism, I realize that what she described the man as doing was actually Magnetization of the water. She said the relief was instant. As she drank the water, the headache just melted away.

There is no limit as to how often or in what quantity you can use the "healing waters."

Magnetized Cotton

For this you need a roll of absorbent cotton such as you can get in a drugstore.

Cut a piece about the size of your hand, or the size you might need to cover a specific area—a cut or abrasion, for example.

Then Magnetize the cotton by either (1) holding it between your two palms and doing a "contact" Short Circuit on it, (2) holding it in your negative hand and holding your positive palm an inch or so above the cotton, or (3) laying the cotton down on some surface and Putting In to it for several minutes. I prefer the third option, but do what comes naturally to mind.

Bandages and band-aids can be magnetized in this way, also, before application.

Dolores Krieger has found that cotton Magnetized in this way will keep its effectiveness indefinitely.

10

PASS IT ON

Did you know that at one time in this country Magnetic Healing was so widespread and popular that even the most sober practitioners predicted that it would replace all other forms of treatment in a few decades? Tens of thousands flocked to Dr. Weltmer's Institute in Nevada, Missouri, where it was common to treat *four hundred* people a day. And that was only one center.

Today, Magnetic Therapy is virtually unknown.

What happened?

The same thing that happened to the great movement of Anton Mesmer: greed and "professionalism." People opened up offices and "clinics," kept their "healing secrets" to themselves (or taught them for a high price to students—usually sworn to secrecy—who in their turn did the same), and charged people for what the patients—or their family members—could have done themselves. I have a book that claims to be a *guide* for Magnetic healers. It is 125 pages long, but only a little over five pages is instruction, and that instruction is so poorly and sketchily given that no one could apply it. And that was the author's intention—to make money on a book, yet not tell would-be competitors how to "do the stuff"! This self-seeking mentality has caused a great knowledge to almost be lost. And it *is*, as I have said, virtually unknown.

Dr. Mesmer lamented: "The advantages and the singular nature of this system was responsible, some years ago, for the eagerness of the public to grasp the first hopes which I held out; and it is by perverting them that envy, presumption and incredulity have in a very short space of time succeeded in relegating them to the status of illusions, causing them to fall into oblivion."

Even worse—because it is deception—some people have used these natural principles of healing, but dressed them up with the titles of "psychic healing" or "spiritual healing," while touting their "unique gift" as "from God" and giving God "the credit" (though not a cut of the profit, I'll warrant!), even though they know that all their admirers and financial supporters can do the same as they. (The few who don't know this are "plain ignorant," which may in some instances be even worse.)

80

This is truly despicable.

I have spent a great deal of time and money researching and writing this book. Not one penny from this book will ever come to me from this effort. All profit from this book will go into a fund to print more books to help others. But I would like to ask a "profit" from you: apply these principles in your own life and *pass it on*. Help others of your family. Teach them these things. Get more copies of this little book and give them to your friends. Spread the word around. The good you do will benefit both you and me, for our neighbor *is* ourself, and when one is benefited we all gain from it.

At the end of his life, Mesmer wrote: "More important than the obstacles which have been thrown in my way, I have believed it necessary to progress to publish my ideas. I voluntarily surrender my theory to criticism, declaring that I have neither the time nor the desire to reply to it. I have nothing to say to those who are incapable of crediting me with integrity or generosity, and who cannot substitute anything better for that of mine which they seek to destroy.

"I would regard with pleasure any better inspirations which might bring forth sounder, more enlightened principles—some talent better understood than mine, which might discover new facts and perhaps make my doctrine even more beneficial by new conceptions and work. In brief, I wish that someone might go further than I have gone. . . .

"Although I am rather advanced in years, I wish to dedicate my remaining life to the sole practice of a method that I have discovered to be eminently useful in the preservation of my fellowman, in order that hereafter they might not be further exposed to the incalculable hazards of the applications of drugs."

This book is ended. But I pray that it is only the beginning for you and for many others.

God bless you. Pray for me.

FOOTNOTES

1. *Laetrile: Nutritional Control for Cancer with Vitamin B-17*, Glenn D. Kittler, Royal Publications, 1978.

2. *The Grape Cure*, Johanna Brandt, Ehret Literature Publishing Co.

3. *The Master Cleanser*, Stanley Burroughs, P.O. Box 260, Kailua, HI 96374. 1976.

4. Johanna Brandt, author of *The Grape Cure*.

5. *The Health Secrets of a Naturopathic Doctor*, M.O. Garten, D.O., Parker Publishing, 1967.

6. *The Vegetarian's Self-defense Manual*, Richard Bargen, M.D., Theosophical Publishing House, 1979.

7. *Magic: Science of the Future*, Joseph F. Goodavage, Signet, 1976.

8. *Nutrition Almanac*, John D. Kirschmann, McGraw-Hill, 1975.

9. *Diet for a Small Planet*, Frances Moore Lappe, Ballantine Books, 1971.

10. *Recipes for a Small Planet*, Ellen Buchman Ewald, Ballantine Books, 1973.

11. *Warning: Sex May Be Hazardous to Your Health*, Dr. Edwin Flatto, Arco Publishing Company, 1975.

12. *Vital Magnetic Cure: An Exposition of Vital Magnetism by a Magnetic Physician.* Health Research

RECOMMENDED READING

1. *The Therapeutic Touch*, Dolores Krieger, Prentice-Hall, 1979.

2. *The Master Cleanser*, Stanley Burroughs, P.O. Box 260, Kailua, HI 96374. 1976.

3. *Diet for a Small Planet*, Frances Moore Lappe, Ballantine Books, 1971.

4. *Recipes for a Small Planet*, Ellen Buchman Ewald, Ballantine Books, 1973.

5. *The Health Secrets of a Naturopathic Doctor*, M.O. Garten, D.O., Parker Publishing, 1967.

6. *The Vegetarian's Self-defense Manual*, Richard Bargen, M.D., Theosophical Publishing House, 1979.

7. *Warning: Sex May Be Hazardous to Your Health*, Dr. Edwin Flatto, Arco Publishing Company, 1975.

8. *Laetrile: Nutritional Control for Cancer with Vitamin B-17*, Glenn D. Kittler, Royal Publications, 1978.

9. *The Grape Cure*, Johanna Brandt, Ehret Literature Publishing Co.

10. *Nutrition Almanac*, John D. Kirschmann, McGraw-Hill, 1975.

11. The catalog of books on health published by Health Research Associates, Box 70, Mokelumne Hill, CA 95245.

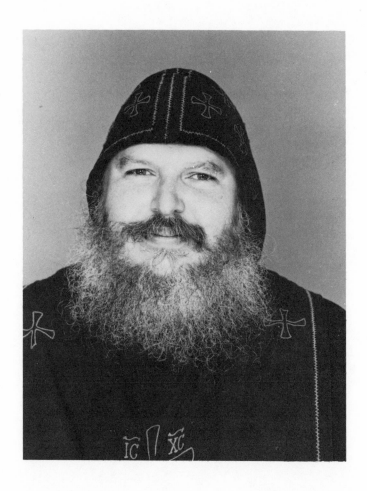

ABBOT GEORGE BURKE, the author of *Magnetic Therapy*, is the founder and head of the Holy Protection Orthodox Monastery in Oklahoma City.

Although his major involvement is in research and writing on the original esoteric wisdom of Christianity, Abbot Burke has been actively involved in the field of drugless therapy for many years and regularly teaches classes in various drugless therapies both in Oklahoma and in other states.